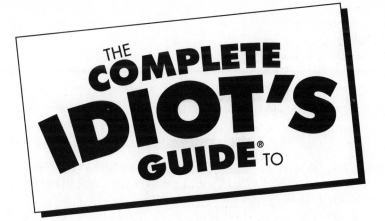

THE COMPLETE IDIOT'S GUIDE® TO

Running Injury-Free

D0973602

by Coach Damon Martin,
with Bob Schaller

ALPHA

A member of Penguin Group (USA) Inc.

ALPHA BOOKS

Published by the Penguin Group

Penguin Group (USA) Inc., 375 Hudson Street, New York, New York 10014, USA

Penguin Group (Canada), 90 Eglinton Avenue East, Suite 700, Toronto, Ontario M4P 2Y3, Canada (a division of Pearson Penguin Canada Inc.)

Penguin Books Ltd., 80 Strand, London WC2R 0RL, England

Penguin Ireland, 25 St. Stephen's Green, Dublin 2, Ireland (a division of Penguin Books Ltd.)

Penguin Group (Australia), 250 Camberwell Road, Camberwell, Victoria 3124, Australia (a division of Pearson Australia Group Pty. Ltd.)

Penguin Books India Pvt. Ltd., 11 Community Centre, Panchsheel Park, New Delhi—110 017, India

Penguin Group (NZ), 67 Apollo Drive, Rosedale, North Shore, Auckland 1311, New Zealand (a division of Pearson New Zealand Ltd.)

Penguin Books (South Africa) (Pty.) Ltd., 24 Sturdee Avenue, Rosebank, Johannesburg 2196, South Africa

Penguin Books Ltd., Registered Offices: 80 Strand, London WC2R 0RL, England

International Standard Book Number: 978-159257-733-0
Library of Congress Catalog Card Number: 2007937307

10 09 08   8 7 6 5 4 3 2

Interpretation of the printing code: The rightmost number of the first series of numbers is the year of the book's printing; the rightmost number of the second series of numbers is the number of the book's printing. For example, a printing code of 08-1 shows that the first printing occurred in 2008.

Printed in the United States of America

Note: This publication contains the opinions and ideas of its authors. It is intended to provide helpful and informative material on the subject matter covered. It is sold with the understanding that the authors and publisher are not engaged in rendering professional services in the book. If the reader requires personal assistance or advice, a competent professional should be consulted.

The authors and publisher specifically disclaim any responsibility for any liability, loss, or risk, personal or otherwise, which is incurred as a consequence, directly or indirectly, of the use and application of any of the contents of this book.

Most Alpha books are available at special quantity discounts for bulk purchases for sales promotions, premiums, fund-raising, or educational use. Special books, or book excerpts, can also be created to fit specific needs.

For details, write: Special Markets, Alpha Books, 375 Hudson Street, New York, NY 10014.

Publisher: *Marie Butler-Knight*
Editorial Director/Acquiring Editor: *Mike Sanders*
Managing Editor: *Billy Fields*
Senior Development Editor: *Phil Kitchel*
Production Editor: *Kayla Dugger*
Copy Editor: *Amy Borrelli*

Cartoonist: *Shannon Wheeler*
Cover Designer: *Bill Thomas*
Book Designer: *Trina Wurst*
Indexer: *Tonya Heard*
Layout: *Ayanna Lacey*
Proofreader: *Mary Hunt*

Contents at a Glance

Contents

Introduction

We all run at some point in our lives. We stop as we get older because we don't have time, we put on some weight, or we hurt ourselves.

It doesn't have to be that way—well, except for the "we all get older" part; we can't change that. But you can keep *feeling* younger, and in better shape, as you get older. And you can do it by running and staying injury-free.

I've coached hundreds of runners and won dozens of titles and Coach of the Year honors during my tenure at NCAA powerhouse Adams State College in Colorado. To have my runners win, they have to be able to run, which means keeping them injury-free. Running, when done properly, extends your life, makes you feel better with more energy and a more fit body, and keeps your heart and muscles in good shape. So let's take that first step into the rest of your life—a more enjoyable, healthier, fulfilling life.

How to Use This Book

I divided this book into five parts to make it more user friendly. All of these chapters apply to anyone who wants to run injury-free—from someone reading this on the couch, to someone who wants to run a local race, and even to those who are already running regularly.

Part 1, "Run for Your Life," explains the proper running form, how the body works when you run, and where the various body parts should and should not be. This part then gets us on the path to a healthy running lifestyle by looking at running as a holistic activity that benefits the mind, body, and even the way you feel about yourself. I walk you through a program called "periodization" that gets you on an injury-free path to steady improvement, and we also set some goals together that make sense and inspire you.

Part 2, "Finding Your Stride," discusses the right fuel for your machine and puts body weight in the proper perspective. Then we'll go through an amazing warm-up and cooldown cycle that gets the most out of each while getting your body ready for this run and the next one. Stretching is a staple of warm-ups, cooldowns, and your overall running diet, and we'll review a whole menu of them. We also get into how much sleep is enough, and how important this underrated part of your life is.

In **Part 3, "Running and Dressing Defensively,"** I will explain everything about footwear—in fact, I'll do everything but try the shoes on for you! Then we'll head out onto your preferred running surface, and discuss every other surface in detail. This part also talks about the weather, when to run, when not to, what to wear, and why hot weather requires proper attire just as much as cold weather. Finally, we'll look at the many risks of the road.

Part 4, "Listen When Your Body Talks," takes you through a veritable alphabet soup of injuries and explains each one. Injuries are like potholes; if you know where they are, you won't step in them. We'll discuss the difference between soreness and actual pain, when you are too sick to run, and when you can run even though you don't feel your best. I also get into how to best treat actual injuries, and offer alternative training and exercises to do until you're ready to really run again.

Extras

Throughout this book, you'll see tons of helpful and informative sidebars that help illustrate a point or caution you to be aware of something.

Watch Your Step _____

These are pieces of advice that will educate you on a common misstep taken by many runners.

Runner Facts _____

These are facts and numbers about the running injury-free lifestyle that extend your knowledge of the sport and help your training.

Road Blocks _____

These keep you on track by avoiding a pitfall that is out there—yet one you can avoid if you are aware of it.

In Their Shoes

These take you out on a run with runners I have coached to show the practical application of a point I have made in the text. These runners sharing their stories with you might be among the better training partners you ever have!

Acknowledgments

Bernard of Chartres said that we are "like dwarfs on the shoulders of giants, so that we can see more than they, and things at a greater distance, not by virtue of any sharpness of sight on our part, or any physical distinction, but because we are carried high and raised up by their giant size."

As I have stood at podiums and accepted awards and trophies during my career, I have never been there alone. Through every victory and defeat and all the accomplishments, I have truly been blessed to stand on the shoulders of giants. The giants in my life are the student athletes who have gone the extra mile to ensure our team's success. Regardless of the sacrifices they faced or the challenges we encountered, each one of them embraced the program and became part of our long green line. I can honestly say that they have given me as much as I was ever able to give them.

My family and community are my other giants. I would like to thank my mom and dad and my brother for always being there for me. And to the coaches in my life who saw something in me that I wasn't always able to see in myself, thank you for your faith in me and for your inspiration. I want to extend a special thank you to the people of the San Luis Valley and my Adams State College family. Your encouragement and support, your cheers and your hugs, have made each year special and helped to lift our program to the absolute top.

Thanks also to my co-author, Bob Schaller, whose guidance and friendship has made this process not only smoother, but more enjoyable as well.

And most important of all, to my wife, Konnie, and two children, Lauren and Tanner, whom I love and thank for their unconditional love and support.

Special Thanks to the Technical Reviewers

The Complete Idiot's Guide to Running Injury-Free was reviewed and edited by experts who either run competitively or worked for a wellness clinic to make sure you are getting good advice that keeps you running smart and injury-free. Special thanks to my runners and coaching staff who have gone the extra mile, and then some, to make sure everything in this book is sound in principle and practice.

Trademarks

All terms mentioned in this book that are known to be or suspected of being trademarks or service marks have been appropriately capitalized. Alpha Books and Penguin Group (USA) Inc. cannot attest to the accuracy of this information. Use of a term in this book should not be regarded as affecting the validity of any trademark or service mark.

Part 1

Run for Your Life

Is there a right way to run? You've seen runners slouched over, runners leaning back, runners taking tiny steps, runners taking mighty strides, and so on. Yes, there's a right way—and a lot of wrong ways. It's time to find out how your body works when you run optimally and safely.

Smart running and training can avoid injuries, and that's what my whole goal is for users of this book. A holistic approach to running will keep us injury-free. Everything we do ties together. Running is a form of health care, so by definition, running done with some thought is going to make your life better.

I'll explain how your body works, how the energy for running is created, and how your heart and lungs will propel you to new levels. I'll also show you how important a good "base" is if you are seeking to improve. Finally, we'll start building a training program based on your goals.

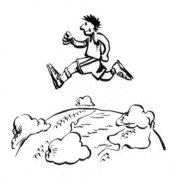

Bodyworks: The Biomechanical Man

In This Chapter

◆ Understanding the mechanics of running to keep yourself injury-free

◆ The keys to proper posture

◆ Avoiding bad habits while developing good ones

◆ The importance of lower leg work to healthy improvement

Understanding your running mechanics is critical if you're going to build a running program that keeps you injury-free. Great running form looks simple—one foot in front of the other—but it takes conscientious effort and practice to develop good bio-mechanics. Having good biomechanics (running form) will help you prevent a slew of common injuries by putting the stress of running on the bones and muscles that are intended to take the beating, and not on parts of your body that aren't.

Be Your Own Best Mechanic

As coaches, we want to make sure that our runners understand how important biomechanics are to how they look and feel, and how utilizing proper form will improve their running as well as keep them injury-free. It is much easier to develop proper form up front; if you don't, it will take consistent work to reprogram your biomechanics.

It is also important to remember that there will be some differences from person to person, so just because you don't look exactly like a track star when you run doesn't necessarily mean that you need to change your running form. We are all built a little differently, and throughout my coaching career I have coached runners of all shapes and sizes. Though they all had their distinctive running styles, the basic principles of biomechanics applied to all of them—and will apply to you as well.

The Upper Body

Do you remember the song that describes how the bones are all connected—"the head bone's connected to the neck bone," and so on? As you develop good running form, it is important to remember this concept. Good running form is a sequential act: if one body part is out of alignment, it is going to affect the other areas of your body and ruin your form.

This can also be demonstrated by Newton's third law of motion: for every action there is an equal and opposite reaction. If you oscillate your shoulders side to side when you run, this will create torque in the hips, which will cause the hips and legs to conversely oscillate as well.

Let me describe the basics of good posture and running form from head to toe.

Head and Neck Position

Hold your head in a neutral position. This will be key to maintaining your overall good posture, which will ultimately determine how efficiently you run. Keeping you head in a natural position with your face relaxed is important. Do not tilt your head forward to look down at your feet; this puts your body in a bad biomechanical position to run efficiently.

Let your eyes direct you. A helpful hint is to scan the horizon; try not to let objects on the horizon bounce too much. This will help you eliminate vertical oscillation in your running style and help you keep a straighter neck and back. Don't allow your chin to jut out.

Shoulders

Keeping your shoulders down and at ease is very important in keeping your upper body relaxed while you run. This sets up the proper alignment for correct running posture.

Keeping your shoulders low and loose, not high and tight, will help you maintain better range of motion with your arms and will prevent your back from becoming tight as well. If your shoulders start to get tight and begin creeping up, shake your arms and rotate your shoulders a few times. This trick often helps the shoulders relax.

Arms, Wrists, and Hands

It is crucial to learn good technique with your arms and hands. Your arm motion impacts several aspects of your running form. Your arms affect your stride length, stride frequency, and your side-to-side oscillation issues. Although running is largely a lower-body activity, your arms provide assistance to your legs.

Start by cupping your hands loosely and keeping them very relaxed. Many young runners clench their fists to try and run faster, but this is just the opposite of what you should do. Keeping them loose and relaxed will reduce the tension that can build up in your shoulders and chest.

Your arms should be bent at the elbow at about a 90-degree angle, as if you were shaking someone's hand. Keep your wrists in the up position, as this will prevent your arms from swaying across the midline of your body; this will further eliminate oscillation of your body. The swinging of your arms will work in conjunction with your leg strides, which will help you to drive your legs forward and backward.

If you feel your hands beginning to clench, use the same trick as you do with your shoulders and shake your hands and arms out to relax them.

Chest

Your chest position is affected by the position of your head and shoulders. With your head up and your eyes looking forward, your chest and back should naturally straighten to let your body run efficiently and effectively. An upright chest position puts your lungs in the best position for optimal breathing.

Runner Facts

Strong abdominals and back muscles work in tandem. Having a strong core will prevent scores of injuries and help you maintain proper running form as you fatigue

This chest position is also best for optimal stride length. If you allow your chest to rotate forward, it will change where your center of mass is, which will in turn change where your foot lands on the ground.

Do not allow yourself to slouch while you run! This can develop quickly into a lazy biomechanical problem that will limit your performance sometime down the road. I give coaching cues to my athletes like "run tall" or "feel like you're being held by a puppeteer." This helps them understand and feel the proper sensation of running tall. Once you have practiced it right over and over, it will become second nature, and you will reap the benefits of a great running form.

The Lower Body

Having good chest posture helps to make sure your hips will also be in the ideal position. If you have done things right thus far, then your hip area should be your center of mass. This is critical to efficient and injury-free running.

Hips and Butt

If your upper body leans too far forward, your center of mass will be in front of your hip area, which will cause you to put your foot further in front of your body and put more stress on the front of your legs, especially the shins. This happens as a result of your pelvis tilting forward as well.

Many times I tell my athletes that they look like they're sitting while running, or like their butt is in a bucket. I tell them to straighten their back and pull their butt in, and don't allow it to stick out. This will reduce pressure on your lower back and put your hips in a better position to allow your legs to do their job.

Legs

Your legs will have lower or higher knee lift depending on the intensity and length of the run. While running long distances, your knee lift doesn't need to be as significant and your stride length doesn't need to be as long. A sprinter needs a pronounced leg lift and a much longer stride, but it is very difficult to maintain these biomechanics in distance running.

It is important to be efficient and economical, as this will allow you to run longer without wasting energy and effort. Your foot should strike the ground directly underneath your body, so that your center of mass is supported all the way to the ground. When your foot impacts the ground, your knee should be slightly flexed so that it can bend naturally on impact. Do not allow your lower leg to extend in front of your knee, as this will increase your chance of having lower leg injuries.

Another part of the running cycle is the recovery phase—the forward swing of the leg. As the leg comes forward, the heel approaches the butt and the knee is in an upward swing. As your thigh reaches the top of its motion, there is a float period. Your forward leg will start to drop, the knee will move downward, the lower leg will unfold at the knee, and your nearly straight leg moves backward toward the ground. If your posture is erect, your foot will strike the ground almost underneath your body. If your foot contacts the ground too far out front of your body, you'll experience braking forces (slowing down).

Ankles, Feet, and Toes

Your foot should strike the ground naturally, and you should only change this motion if it is impeding your ability to run fast or is causing a problem. The most common problem would be severe heel strikers. This form issue causes runners to experience braking forces as the foot is landing too far out in front of the body.

Most runners strike their heel when they run. A smaller number of runners are mid-foot strikers, which can be a good compromise to allow you to run more efficiently and still not get injured. If you strike the ground with your forefoot, you are in the smallest percentage of runners. There are distinct advantages and drawbacks to each style of running.

If you are a heel striker, the biggest benefit to your legs and body is the shock absorption provided as your foot pronates. Normal foot prona-tion provides cushioning for your leg and body as the foot rolls through the heel to the midfoot and off the toe. Although normal pronation—when the foot rolls only slightly inward, which is common—is good, too much of a good thing can turn bad. If you are an overpronater, you increase your risk of injuries to the lower leg and knee. If you are a forefoot striker, then you have only limited pronation because your foot is on the ground less time. This type of movement doesn't afford you the cushioning benefit that pronation provides.

However, if you do run on your forefoot, then you have the ability to produce more power with each stride, which allows you to run faster. Running on your forefoot is powerful, but it's not as efficient as heel and/or midfoot running. Although most runners are heel-to-toe run-ners, it is interesting to note that most world-class distance runners run on their forefoot. Although most elite distance runners are forefoot strikers, this biomechanic style of running is becoming less prevalent, as far fewer marathoners have adopted this style.

Finding Your Form

Adjusting the way you run can be very tedious. If you plan on making any changes to your biomechanics, it is important that you do so very gradually. I believe that most of you will at some point want to increase your fitness, times, and distances, and you will begin to tinker with your form. Be gradual in your approach and use good common sense.

If you decide to change the way your foot strikes the ground, I suggest that, if you are a heel striker, you gradually progress to a midfoot style.

I don't suggest trying to go from heel striker to a forefoot striker; this will severely increase your likelihood of injury. If you are interested in running faster, try the midfoot style and, if you have pain or tightness symptoms, back off the amount of time running with your new style and allow your body more time to adapt.

A Few Basic Drills

To develop a better running form and strengthen your lower legs, do these exercises a couple times a week. Even if you're in your off season, it takes a lot of patience to change your running form, so don't get discouraged. Changing your biomechanics takes time, but it will pay off when you're running faster and staying healthy.

In order to break the running motion down and isolate certain movements so you can work on improving your technique, I have listed some running form drills. These are called the *ABC drills*, and they should be done as a set; each one addresses a different aspect of your running motion.

The A drill involves lifting your leg and bringing your thigh close to parallel to the ground. Your leg is bent at the knee at an approximate 90-degree angle. As you raise your leg, you will dorsiflex your foot, or pull your toes upward toward your shin. While doing this, your arms should be executing normal running motion. Once your raised leg reaches near parallel, your leg comes to a stop and actively returns downward to the ground. Once this leg returns to the ground, your opposite leg will repeat this same motion. The whole drill looks like an exaggerated up and down running motion.

The B drill begins exactly like the A drill. Once your thigh reaches the near parallel position and the downward motion of the leg happens, your lower leg unfolds at the knee joint, bringing the leg to a nearly straight (slightly bent) position. Your foot is still flexing upward, with the toes still pulled to the shin. As your foot nears the ground, your foot should plantar flexion into the ground. The arms should repeat the same motion as in the A drill.

The final drill is the C drill. This drill begins by bringing the heel of your foot up to or near your buttocks. Your leg is folded at the knee with the heel of your foot near your butt, then your foot returns to the ground. (We often call this drill "butt kicks.") Repeat this motion over and over again.

Watch Your Step

As you become adapted to these drills and distances, you can increase your distance to 35 to 50 meters.

The ABC drills should progress from walking to skipping slowly, to medium-intensity skipping, to finally skipping quickly or running. You may want to begin by doing the ABC drills for three sets: slow for about 25 to 30 meters, then medium for 25 to 30 meters, and then fast for 25 to 30 meters.

Good running form is an art, not an exact science. Consider all the parts of your body and how they relate to one another before you attempt to adjust or change. You don't need or want to look like the runner next door; just incorporate the basics and then build the small things into your running plan and you will notice an improvement.

How do you know if you have good running form? Most of us can't look in a mirror as we're running down the street! I suggest running on a treadmill in a fitness club every now and then and observing yourself in the mirror. Do you see anything that needs adjusting?

Another idea is to have someone videotape you while running in a park or around the track. If you notice anything in the pictures, incorporate some changes into your form. Remember to keep them simple and gradual. Too much change too fast is a sure way to get an injury.

The Least You Need to Know

◆ Everyone is unique—let's find what works for you.

◆ Your core is a key, but often overlooked, part of injury-free running.

◆ Strengthening your lower legs helps you avoid injuries.

◆ The idea that everything is connected is completely true in running—keep it in mind.

Chapter 2

Injury-Free: A Holistic Approach

In This Chapter

- How running coincides with everything else you do in life
- Why you should listen to your body
- Why you should consider running a form of health care
- How running provides a longer, better life

"Taking the first step"—four very simple yet very hard words. Most of us set out to improve our fitness because we want to lead a healthier life. Some of us come to this point because of a major health change: we have a condition, injury, or illness that has given us new incentives. Or maybe we simply realize that living healthier will improve our quality of life.

Whatever the reasons, you are here. And I want you to be successful in your endeavor of running injury-free. I believe that looking at running and life in a holistic manner is your best bet for staying healthy while meeting or exceeding your running goals.

Off and Running

According to Lao-tzu, a Chinese philosopher, "A journey of a thousand miles begins with a single step." As you begin any journey in life, it's important to start with a well-thought-out plan, a good road map, or a strong philosophy about where you are and where you want to go.

Knowing where you are trying to go helps you stay on track when detours come up out of nowhere. I call them detours because calling them roadblocks can make them seem insurmountable and often cause people to quit. I don't want you to feel like you ever need to quit your running program. Among the many positives of running is the fact that you can do it for most of your life, and it is relatively inexpensive in almost any part of the world.

It's more than okay to adjust your training when you need to, but it's not healthy or wise to wander aimlessly without a training plan. This guide will provide you with the tools you need to get fit, stay fit, and avoid injuries along the way. I'll share my philosophy on preventing and treating running-related injuries, which I believe will help you avoid the mistakes my athletes and I have made and learned from over the past 18 years. Many of these mistakes were in overdoing it, running-wise; and underdoing it, recovery-wise.

Running as Part of Your Health Plan

Running is one of the simplest ways to get in shape and remain healthy. Your running program should help you achieve lifetime fitness and wellness, as well as self-control and discipline. Discipline is a trait we all could use more of, but if you truly lack discipline, it will be difficult for you to make significant advances and stay injury-free. Self-discipline is as key to successful training as the running itself.

When it comes to improving your health, you should be a consummate student. It is imperative that we all take a more active approach to improving our fitness and preventing some of society's biggest killers. It is amazing when you consider the health benefits of exercising even just a few hours each week. Most of the focus of our current medical system is on caring for the sick and injured and nursing them back to normal health, rather than being dedicated to prevention and health. When you want to get healthy and begin a training program, you are often on your own in finding the right methods.

As you begin to work on lifetime fitness, focus on developing a comprehensive training program that incorporates all the key elements for your success: nutrition, sleep, rest, mental and spiritual well-being, as well as the many therapies that can help you recover from stresses, strains, and even injuries.

Why Holistic Is Important

Consistently using a comprehensive and holistic approach to injury-free running will not only help you prevent injuries but will also reduce your time off if and when you suffer them. I often come across athletes who don't care about proper rest or nutrition, or don't follow patient, disciplined therapies for recovering from an injury. They're often young and inexperienced, so they think they're invincible and that cutting one workout short or taking an extra day off will do it.

For some, that may be true—for now! But for most of us, especially as we mature (I like that word better than "age"), our bodies change or our old, bad habits catch up with us and we need to do things differently to get a good result.

Taking a holistic approach to preventing injuries and healing injuries basically means devising a comprehensive plan to utilize any and all resources and training to help you reach your goals: a healthy state physically, mentally, and emotionally, and an improved quality of life as well. This holistic approach requires you to take a look at your whole lifestyle, including physical, nutritional, environmental, emotional, social, and spiritual influences. The big-picture perspective will allow you to make more informed decisions, and just maybe you'll try a new approach to a nagging or reoccurring problem.

In Their Shoes

I would like to share a story with you from the 2001 World Track and Field Championships. I went to Edmonton, Canada, in August 2001 to cheer on one of my athletes who was competing in the 800 meters. It was an unbelievable experience to be around so many talented, hard-working athletes, coaches, and medical personnel. I made it a point to go to the practice track every day to watch different athletes train and coaches coach, but several of my most profound memories were from hanging around the medical tent and witnessing the range of therapies athletes were receiving.

One day I witnessed a world-class sprinter receiving electro-stimulation through acupuncture needles inserted into his upper hamstring/lower buttocks area. I had heard of acupuncture for years, but this was my first time actually seeing it done. I was even more amazed when the physiotherapist began to hook electrical clips to groupings of acupuncture needles to stimulate the muscle tissue deeper than other methods could reach.

I was skeptical of these treatments, because I had never heard or known of anyone who had received this therapy. I was curious and struck up a conversation with the physiotherapist and the athlete, and was surprised to learn that electro-acupuncture was developed in China around 1934. This particular athlete had chronic pain and spasms in the upper hamstring/lower buttocks area and had tried numerous other therapies. I vividly remember the athlete saying how many things he had tried; nothing else worked, yet this therapy had given him significant relief, thus allowing him to return to world-class sprinting.

I'm not saying this therapy will work for all injuries, but the important lesson is that there are therapies that aren't mainstream that can give you relief and help you return to running earlier than traditional methods.

Get Better Faster, Smarter

I'm always interested in alternative treatments—particularly ones that I have seen work. A traditional medical provider's first response to any injury or illness is usually to suggest complete rest or time off. This may be best for some injuries, but others may heal in half the time with alternative medicines or therapies. If you don't take the time to find the root cause of the injury (overtraining, undertraining, and so on), you're doomed to repeat the same mistake over and over.

Once this cycle gets going, runners often become frustrated and end up quitting the exercise they love. Don't fall into this trap! Develop your comprehensive plan and adjust your training program to help you stay on the road and off the exam table. Keep an open mind as you learn more about the different elements of training and lifestyle habits that affect your ability to remain healthy and fit.

One common difference that the holistic approach can provide runners is the use of alternative medicines and treatments. Alternative medicine is simply medical techniques that are not as well known or accepted by the majority of medical practitioners. Many of these techniques include noninvasive, nonpharmaceutical treatments such as the use of herbs, acupuncture, homeopathy, and many others. Recent surveys have shown that more Americans are aware of herbs and their benefits than ever before. I believe that this knowledge base is helping these treatments become more mainstream and more available to everyday runners.

Running *Is* Health Care

Most of us are running to improve our total health, but many of our injuries occur as a result of doing more than we need to. Because of our obsessive, competitive nature, we shift the focus from health and fitness to competition; this is where staying healthy becomes more complicated.

We are all tempted at one time or another to take the short path to immediate success. It is vital to remember that true running success happens as a result of doing the process correctly and staying consistent in our approach. More often than not, I see runners try to cheat the system by skipping steps of adaptation. This may help you achieve one or two seasonal best marks, only to be followed by an injury or the need for a long rest.

Getting into shape is a long process, but the benefits are also long lasting. As you work to get in shape, it's important to lay a foundation for long-term health. This mentality will help you stay true to doing things the right way. It all fits together: lifestyle, nutrition, hydration, biomechanics, periodization, motivation, stretching, weight training, rest, and recovery.

How Running Ties It All Together

Many runners begin running for the physical exercise and a greater sense of well-being, only to learn that running is also a great way to meditate. It becomes a regular part of your routine and everyday spiritual practice. As you gain greater confidence in your running capabilities, you might consider joining a running group or trying some of the local running clubs training runs. Many people who thought they weren't good enough to run with others progress to wanting to run a couple of local road races. I believe that most runners benefit as much psychologically from running as physiologically. Recognize the true payback of an overall running and training program and then pursue this endeavor with the knowledge that injury-free running will provide lifelong fitness and better quality of life.

To establish your personal fitness goals, think about what you intend to accomplish. Pick an audacious goal, something way out there such as competing in a local 10k race, improving your individual time by 10 percent, or dropping that weight you've been carrying. Then set several intermediate goals to give you something to aim for and several opportunities to celebrate your accomplishments in stages. Taking the time to recognize your advancements will give you a more positive attitude and help you reach those big goals that are waiting out there for you.

Once you set your goal and establish a timeline, begin developing your training program. Chapter 3 on periodization will be your guide. It breaks the training period into several subsections and lays the foundation for planning the various components of your program.

By taking a systematic approach, you'll greatly reduce the opportunity for injury. You'll also have checks and balances to prevent you from over- or undertraining as you strive to improve your health. In my experience, overtraining is the biggest reason for injury, and a big contributor when runners don't reach their intended goals or don't reach them on time.

I think of running as a way of life. This is very different from the person who sees it as work. To me it is a way to manage your health without much outside intervention. People who improve their fitness need less medical care, they stay more agile and flexible as they age, they burn off a lot of the physical symptoms of stress, and the psychological benefits of endorphins released during exercise (runner's high) are well documented. So regardless of whether you run to stay fit or if you stay fit to run—*RUN!* It will improve both your quality and quantity of life!

In Their Shoes

When you've coached for years, you develop your own way of identifying types of runners. There are a group of very special athletes that I always call the "1-percenters." They are the ones that, whatever the odds of an injury or accident occurring, it always happens to them.

I have coached only a few 1-percenters, but needless to say, I just never knew what would happen next. One young lady that I coached for many years took the prize for weird accidents; she seemed destined to find (accidentally) any looming hazard. Our team would go out for a training run on a seemingly clear path or trail and before we knew it, she had found a pothole to step in or maybe a stump to run into.

On one unfortunate run, an entire group of runners made it around this partial wire fence with no fanfare, but of course our 1-percenter ran right in the wire, slicing her leg right above the knee. Ten stitches made for an interesting scare. Once that had sufficiently healed and she was back to training, she opted for rollerblading as a cross-training workout. As fate would have it, she fell and broke her jaw. She trained diligently with her mouth wired shut for six weeks, all the while subsisting on nothing but a liquid diet. When she did finally make it back to competition, she had the horrible luck of falling on the last water barrier in a major steeplechase race. The fall cost her the win and injured her leg and knee.

I use this 1-percenter as an example that sometimes things just don't go our way. You may be a 1-percenter or maybe you know one, but the key is to keep a positive attitude and get right back on that horse that threw you. This particular young lady earned many All-American honors as well as helped her team to multiple national team titles. Her attitude always allowed her to overcome obstacles when many others would have packed it in. If you're a 1-percenter, then it's imperative you keep a great outlook, and you will be a stronger person as a result of it.

A Grave Reminder

When I first began my career, I focused more on health education and injury prevention before I moved 100 percent into coaching. I used to give my classes an illustration of quality of life as it relates to a holistic and comprehensive fitness program.

Imagine a cemetery with two headstones next to one another, of men born in the same year. The first headstone reads: "Born 1900, Died

1960, Buried 1980." The second reads: "Born 1900, Died and Buried 1980."

The difference between these two men is the quality of life they lived. While one became unhealthy, unable to enjoy even the simplest excursion or event, the other lived life fully to the end. You see, the first one was a smoker, never did a day of exercise in his life, and ate nothing but fast food. The other man followed a healthy lifestyle plan, eating the right foods and exercising at least five days a week. He remained fit and agile until the very last day of his life.

Sometimes we measure life in years of living; I truly believe we should measure life in years of quality living. If your life were measured in quality versus quantity, how old would you be?

The Least You Need to Know

- Running is part of a healthy lifestyle, not just a sport.

- Running is something that not only lasts a lifetime, but makes a lifetime last longer.

- Listen to coaches and read books, but most of all, listen to your body—it will tell you what it needs.

- Weight loss and being in overall good shape is tied to both eating right and exercise, not just one or the other.

Chapter 3

Setting Goals and Planning Your Training

In This Chapter

- ◆ The process and phases of periodization
- ◆ Why the base phase is so important
- ◆ Why the step method helps runners stay healthy and reach goals
- ◆ How taking a break after big gains can keep you on track to even bigger goals

One of the better aspects of running is that runners don't usually reach their peak until they are 30, or at least in their late 20s. Most of the world's best distance runners are in their 30s; and there are world-class runners even older than that. In fact, if you run local road races, you see senior citizens keeping a good pace. That's the beauty of running: though it's a sport predicated on time, it is timeless.

Running is a long-term activity, and athletes don't reach their peak until they've put in years of building their base; honing their form, muscles, and tendons; and understanding both their bodies and running. You don't just become a better runner overnight. If you train smart and avoid injuries, you can run for the rest of your life.

It All Starts with a Good Base

Since the beginning of the 1970s here at Adams State College, we have won 32 NCAA Cross-Country Championships between the men's and women's programs. That is a phenomenal number if you consider that there is only one championship cross-country meet per year. When coaches and athletes ask me what I believe is the secret to that success, I always cite periodization and proper peaking as one of our keys.

These concepts of peaking cycles and periodization, which means reaching a goal (peak) by breaking down the training needed into phases, directs your training program toward the ultimate goal of running the fastest time at the most important meet. You hear about it in politics and professional sports: it's all about peaking at the right time.

I began the 1994 cross-country season with a young but dedicated group of young women. I could see their potential, but there was virtually no high-level cross-country experience in any of them. They ranged from a converted 400/800-meter runner in her first year of cross-country to an unproven junior college transfer I accepted into the program as a favor for a friend of mine from California.

We began the season as a middle-of-the-pack team in most races. I spent the first half of the season trying to get the team into college running shape before we really began any serious high-level running. I noticed week to week how their strength improved and how their confidence grew. I had this wild thought in the back of my head that by the end of the season we might surprise some people and finish better than most fans thought we could.

We progressed through August and September and into the high-intensity and peaking phases of the season with the athletes responding very favorably. Once the base training had been laid, the intensity and peaking components seemed to be coming together. We finished our conference meet in second place behind a very strong Western State

College team (our primary foe during my tenure here) and then moved into a very strong regional competition. We continued to improve, and some of the athletes were showing signs of surprising strength and determination; again we finished second to Western State.

As we made our way to the national cross-country meet, I knew our team was ready to give a tremendous effort. The workouts showed me that their fitness was reaching its highest point of the year—but when you line up at a really big meet like nationals, it can be incredibly intimidating for even experienced college runners, let alone these novices.

We started the race in good position and as the race progressed, we looked stronger and stronger. The girls began feeding off each other's performances, strength, and determination. They could truly feel the peaking process was working for them. As the race continued, they found themselves near the front of the pack. We ended up winning the national championship that day. Ironically, it was the only meet this team won the entire year.

As I reflect on how periodization and peaking can affect the outcome of a season, I always think back to how that particular team responded to the different phases of training. Their progress was one of the finest improvements and accomplishments in our rich history.

Periodization: A Long Word for Breaking Down Goals

Periodization is a fancy word for proper planning of your training. I consider it a truly fundamental piece of knowing how and when to work and train so you're ready when you choose a race or a fitness goal. Even if you don't plan on racing in some elite road race, periodization will help you see improvements in your training and your mental engagement, and the boost you get from seeing results will demonstrate that running can be a lot more fun than just 20 minutes per day on the same old trail or treadmill.

Periodization helps me structure my team's workouts and prepare our runners to peak at the proper times of the year. This planning will allow you to organize your training program to consistently achieve optimal results without overtraining. Overuse injuries are typically the number-one cause of injuries with athletes. By planning your training over your season or goal period, you can avoid the pitfalls of overuse injuries and still peak at the right time.

I believe in the good old five Ps: *proper planning prevents poor performance!* When planning for your ultimate goal, step back and look at the big picture of your training program. What is your ultimate goal? Is it a race? A personal best time? A certain body weight? Regardless of your goal, without a proper plan you can wander aimlessly. Bad planning can also lead to injuries and illness, disrupting your path toward your goals and setting back your personal health.

The Great Pyramid

I truly believe that 95 percent of great performances happen as a result of doing things right, having a formula, and following steps and procedures. Basically, they are designed and well-executed plans. In order to have great running performances, you must follow a series of preparations that build on one another.

This pyramid is a design that first requires you to build a foundation of physical fitness. The base of fitness will allow you to transition to the next step successfully. Once you have attained adequate physical fitness, then you begin to focus on developing the technical aspects of your running. After these two factors have been firmly established, you will then add tactical preparation to your training program.

And finally, your focus will move to the psychological preparation of your development as a runner. As you progress through these stages, you will find that the better job you do in laying each step down, the easier it becomes to develop the next training factor.

Getting Started the Right Way

The basis of all great athletic performances is your physical preparation. If you have ever heard that 90 percent of a good performance is mental, well, that's certainly not true for endurance runners. You must have a sound training base to stay healthy and perform well in practices and in competition. As you develop your base, your confidence will grow as your fitness improves. As you prepare for racing, then you can focus more on mental factors that will assist you in reaching your goals.

As I begin planning my seasonal workouts for each of my athletes, I look at where they are and what their goals are. I then begin to formulate their training from the end to the beginning. It is important to plan this way to ensure that you have enough time to accomplish all the things that you want to get done in order to run that personal record (PR) or reach that elusive goal. Divide your time into periods or "phases," and set short-, medium-, and long-term goals, preparing for your ultimate goal every step of the way. One benefit of doing it this way is that you don't let things get by you that you meant to work on; therefore, you can fit it all into your plan.

Whenever I start a program, the first step is always setting a series of goals—that drives the program, setting a tone of how and when I'm going to do certain things and how I am going to get the athletes where they need to be in a certain amount of time. Ultimately, we have to figure out what's best for each athlete, but certainly one goal is to choose a path that doesn't lead to injuries. Once you injure yourself, your plan is at least interrupted and might even have to be mostly or completely rethought.

Over the years, I have seen many athletes do the same exact training year after year and not understand why they aren't improving. My goal is to help you understand the basics of developing a well-rounded, progressive plan that will allow you to stay healthy, injury-free, and, of course, race fast and far.

Once you establish your goal, identify the time frame in which your peak needs to occur. Knowing your ending date and starting date will allow you to put together your training plan properly. I know it seems awkward to do it this way, but trust me: for this process, the end is really the beginning.

You will need to understand how your body adapts to the different types of training and levels of adaptation. If you're working to improve your flexibility, you can make fairly steady improvements day to day until you reach a plateau point. At that point, when you are working at speed, your adaptation process will slow a little, becoming more week to week. Strength adaptation occurs more on a month-to-month basis, and endurance adaptation happens year to year. Keep in mind that great increases in endurance take time and in order to stay injury-free, you should not rush this normal adaptation process.

Break It Down to Basics

Being an endurance athlete takes incredible patience and dedication. The physical work and training process is very rewarding, but staying with it is the secret for lifelong fitness. Remember when your parents told you that anything worth having was worth working for? That old adage certainly applies to this situation. Because of the long-term commitment endurance running requires, you will want to make every effort to do the training the right way and stay injury-free.

The following chart shows the step method, a series of three steps up with one step down. This simple stair-step chart shows the relationship between increasing stress (running volume and/or running intensity) over increments of time (adaptation). The step method is a form of making calculated improvements and represents the relationship between improvement and time. The height of the step measures the increase in stress, such as moving your volume of mileage up by 10 percent or running an interval 3 percent faster than the previous phase of interval training. The width represents the amount of time that it will take you to adapt to this new stress.

This chart shows how the step method looks visually as time passes and you increase stress (mileage and/or intensity).

For example, in your first three weeks of running, you were to run 20 miles per week. Then, during your second phase of three weeks, you increased the mileage to 25 miles per week. How much time does it take your body to adjust to this increased level? In most cases, it will take 28 to 31 days, or about four weeks. This represents one step (height and width) on the chart. Now if you have previously trained at some higher mileage level (say 50 miles per week) and are just returning to running after a short time off, you could start at 20 miles per week, go up in shorter intervals, and adjust much faster. Once you reach the level where your body was previously used to, then any major adjustment in volume (stress) will require the 28 to 31 days to fully adjust.

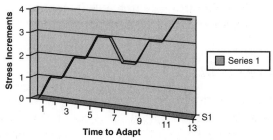

Step method.

Overload, But in a Good Way

Another concept I would like to share with you is the law of overload. Increasing either your volume or intensity will put increased stress on your entire body (muscles, bones, cardiovascular system, pulmonary system, and so on). Your initial physiological reaction to this increase will be fatigue. This sometimes feels as if you are losing fitness, but it's just part of the process of adaptation. When you allow your body ample time to recover from your increases in work (running), your physiological systems will adapt and allow you to reach higher fitness levels.

This is a key point where you can't get discouraged. You might find yourself tired and sore, with a growing desire to reach for the remote instead of your running shoes, but don't give in. Keep the faith and you will be amazed at how your body will adapt; you will build strength and fitness, and that fatigue will fade away.

It is imperative that any increases (volume or intensity) you add must be done consistently and methodically to prevent your body from overuse injuries. An increase of 3 percent is somewhat the norm when working with intensity, and 5 to 10 percent increases are the norm when working with volume. Some programs call for bigger jumps but will put you at a much higher risk of injury. I suggest you stick with the recommended standards (I still use these with my team) of improvement.

Another way to think of this is if you can run an all-out mile in six minutes and you begin your interval training (mile repeats) at 85 percent of your max speed for the mile. This equates to running at 7:03 per interval mile. During the next cycle of your training, increase your intensity to 88 percent of your max speed, or 6:49 per mile. In your third cycle of interval training, move your intensity to 91 percent of your max speed, or 6:35 for the mile.

This example shows you how to reasonably increase your intensity in the interval component of your training plan. Increases that are too aggressive create unstable adaptation and put you at high risk for injury. Increases that are too small don't bring you the results or improvements you are seeking.

Although I see runners who increase their intensity too fast, I believe that even more runners make the same type of mistake with volume. Every fall when our cross-country runners report, there are always two or three athletes who didn't follow the training I laid out for them at the beginning of the summer. And not only did they not run, but they're afraid to tell me! So they make their best effort to jump into the full-volume workout, and will usually last a week to a week and a half before they have some sort of injury.

It's not wise to jump in or overdo training, even when you're behind where you want to be. This will only make the problem worse. Follow the 5 percent/10 percent rule—maybe a little higher if you are a more experienced runner—to ensure stable progress.

As I mentioned earlier, it normally takes the body 28 to 31 days to physiologically adapt to any new stress or exercise you place upon it. This adaptation does not happen in a linear way; you don't adapt an exact 3.3 percent each day for 30 days. Your greatest adaptation occurs during the beginning of new stress: 70 percent in the first 9 to 10 days, then 20 percent more in the next 9 to 10 days, and finally the last 10 percent adaptation happens over the last 9 to 10 days. This again shows the importance of staying on track. Once you complete the first two phases of adaptation, you are 90 percent of our way to being adapted to the new level of training.

Here at Adams State, I change the stress for my workouts once every three weeks. This is before the runners are 100-percent adapted to their increased stress. I usually only allow my runners to adapt to 90 to 92 percent of the new stress during each adaptation phase. This allows me to maximize their improvement by getting the biggest part of adaptation during each phase of the adaptation process; I look at this as focusing on the big money and not worrying about the change. But I caution you not to change any sooner than this. Changing intensities quicker than this will eventually lead to unstable adaptation and erratic performances.

You may learn that your body adapts better by using the whole 28 to 31 days, and individual variance can change depending on how quickly your body adapts to volume and/or intensity increases. If you need the full 31 days to adapt and adjust before you move on to another phase, then by all means take it. You know your body better than anyone, so pay attention to the signs of adaptation so you can recognize how fast you are progressing and re-evaluate the plan if you need to. The warning signs associated with adaptation include more-than-normal fatigue, a higher-than-normal basal heart rate for several days in a row, and being unable to maintain the quality of your workouts for no other apparent reason.

Every runner's situation is different. If you're a veteran runner looking to improve your time, your experience adapting to new levels of stress (increased volume) will be completely different from a runner who's had six months of training experience.

> **Runner Facts**
>
> Several factors influence whether you adapt to increased stress faster or slower than the norm. They include genetic makeup, health status, years of running, resting patterns, nutrition, and overall fitness. If you are concerned with this process, you should evaluate the controllable factors and make any necessary changes.

Recovery, Restoration, and Adaptation

Coaches are notorious for paying incredible attention to workouts and ignoring other significant issues in your overall improvement. If you are running extremely hard, then equal attention must be paid to making sure you fully recover from this exertion.

If you do a hard speed session, it will take the central nervous system 48 to 72 hours to fully recover, so you'll need that much time between one hard workout and the next. Otherwise you will be overstressing your central nervous system and increasing the likelihood of an injury.

That doesn't mean you can't work out; you can enjoy a very easy couple days of running or cross-training.

As you increase volume or intensity, you are adding stress that your body's not used to. This increased stress actually decreases your physical fitness as you tire. With proper rest, your body will start to adapt, which will allow your body to return to your old fitness level. By repeating this cycle, you will teach you body to adapt to your new stresses, thus helping you reach new levels of fitness.

If your running program is too easy, then you will not stress your body enough to produce relevant adaptation. If your running program is extremely difficult, you may spend an inordinate amount of time in the fatigue stage and barely get back to your old fitness level.

I have seen some runners' fitness diminish as they work themselves too hard by believing in the old adage: if a little is good, then more must be better. This philosophy can sometimes be true, but everyone adapts a little differently, so don't overdo it in any one particular workout or phase of training.

A big part of becoming successful is knowing where you are in this adaptation process at all times. If you are still fatigued, then you should either have another easy day or take the day off. If you are fully adapted to your current running workouts, then it is time to add a new stress (running stress, that is!).

Shhh! Listen to Your Body

Another part of periodization, in terms of injury prevention, is that when you add volume and intensity, it creates fatigue. So as you add intensity or volume, you actually feel less fit at first. Then, with proper rest and nutrition, you rise to a higher level. If you don't repeat the stress or increase it, this leads to involution, or falling back or even declining back to the old fitness level.

Age and initial fitness level really do matter. If you're coming back from an injury such as knee surgery, you'll be able to move through the adaptation period at a far different rate than someone who just took two weeks to rest. Don't misunderstand the body's response to anesthesia and/or being sedentary—they both zap your energy and stamina, and you may need some extended time to adapt to your running program. You must proceed thoughtfully and not get down on yourself if you need a longer period before moving on. Listen to your body and do what it tells you. It is truly the best determinant of how much and how often to train.

Applying Cycles, Setting Goals

In the running world, we measure periods of time in phases and cycles. As you apply the step method of physiological adaptation to your running program, you need to understand microcycles and macrocycles. A microcycle represents a time period of 3 to 14 days. I like to use seven days, since most people can understand a one-week period. A macrocycle represents two to six microcycles; I typically incorporate three microcycles (three weeks) in each macrocycle. These measurements of time are the building blocks of a training program that peaks at just the right phase.

When I am preparing for a cross-country season, our peaking goal is the national cross-country meet in late November. I send each runner a summer training schedule in early June, to give the team a 12-week base training phase before we even begin the season. The true training begins in late August, and we will have four macrocycles of three microcycles (three weeks), or an overall program of 12 weeks.

To apply these time cycles to your situation, pick your target point. Will it be the Chicago marathon in the fall, or do you just want to peak in early December and have your transition or off-period over the holidays, with a new starting date after the new year?

Once you set this date, lay out a base period, a higher-intensity training period, and a peaking cycle. Following all these, you will need to rest and recover.

Two Steps Forward and One (Slight) Step Back

A strange twist in this training improvement process is the element of declining in either training volume or intensity. This element does not show up the same way in other sports, but once every three cycles you will need to reduce a component of your training—either lower your mileage or run fewer sets of timed intervals. This allows your body to overcompensate and "catch up" on recovery, then reach for higher levels of fitness.

I have found that the best and safest improvements happen as you take two or three steps forward and then one slight step back in the training process. Most runners worry that this slight step back in training will cause them to lose fitness, but don't worry about taking the step back. It will allow for greater adaptation to occur and is a big part of your overall training plan. It will keep you on track and injury-free.

Because of the obsessive nature of runners, I have seen athletes make the mistake of running hard just for the sake of running hard. They see themselves moving ahead and improving, maybe running faster times, and fall into the trap of believing that the only way they will keep improving is to keep training at harder and harder levels. The result is a higher potential for injury.

Think of a set of building blocks. If you only ever build straight up, the tower will become unstable and tip over. In running, taking steps back in your training every three or four weeks moves you back down the tower of blocks and lets you add more foundation to the tower that represents your training. This strong and fortified base is your foundation to injury-free running and great performances, allowing your tower to reach even greater heights.

For your own training program, consider what your regular phases of training will be. Let's say you build up to 50 to 55 miles per week. Every third week, consider reducing your mileage to 45 miles. Or, if reducing mileage isn't the way you want to handle the step down, slow your interval or training period for one or two workouts.

Trying to understand the big picture of the training process can be difficult, but if you break down each concept, it begins to make sense. Way too often, runners will begin their new program far too aggressively, only to end up quitting. Just about the time their physiological systems are beginning to adapt to the new stress of running, they often become frustrated and pack it in. Members of our community frequently ask me how to start a new fitness program and/or go about losing weight. The best advice that I can give at first is to start a program that you will stick with for years to come. This includes being smart and not overdoing it at the beginning, and sticking it out for the first 30 days. Then and only then can you make a good decision of what it feels like to run and be successful and injury-free.

In Their Shoes

As the season goes on and the intensity increases, I am sometimes faced with runners who don't want to slow down. They feel themselves improving and gaining strength and momentum, and their limited understanding of physiology prevents them from trusting the system.

Sometimes they push to the point that a cold or abnormal fatigue sets in. I then make them rest. (And I do mean *make*—like when you make a child stop something.) I insist they back off and let their body heal and sometimes even use some scare tactics about how this cold will turn into something much worse if they don't take care of themselves. Then they feel better, get healthy, and—lo and behold—their performance jumps up a notch. I always stop and make a point of showing them what rest did, how it changed their course and impacted their overall training. As athletes go through multiple training and peaking cycles, they learn to understand and trust the process.

But what about that rare individual who just won't rest or follow any commonsense guidelines? I've coached a few of those, too. One young man from Texas just couldn't or wouldn't trust the system. He believed he knew better and insisted on working beyond the program limits. He would finish the college workout and then go out and run additional miles. He might bag a race (run really poorly) on purpose because he believed that the next week's race would go better because he would be rested. It didn't turn out that way. More often than not, his race performances were erratic and far below his potential. But most unfortunate is that he got hurt. The overuse injuries would creep up, and any chance of true personal improvement was gone.

I tell you this story not because I think I have the only true training program, but to encourage you to really follow whatever sound training program you get, whether you read about it here or on the Internet, or get it from a coach or running friend. Don't try to go out and supplement the mileage during a planned rest period. Don't jog or race above or below your planned interval times. The only person who really gets negatively affected is you, and usually an injury is in your near future.

Watch Your Density

There are many ways to measure or quantify training. You can measure the amount of miles or kilometers you run, and you can measure calisthenics by repetitions (volume) or weight lifted. When you are dealing with intensity, you can measure it by the percentage of max effort or max heart rate. Density is another component—that is, how many times we repeat an exercise, how hard the set is, and how often we repeat that throughout a week.

Density is very important to stay in tune with your body. This is how many hard training cycles you will do over a particular block. You have to allow for proper recovery. Say you do a 30-minute aerobic run; to fully recover from this run, you might need just four to six hours (if you did a light run). Make sure to stay well hydrated and spend time resting post-run.

> **Watch Your Step**
>
> Interval training can be highly effective—there is no doubt about that—but you have to allow days to recover from it, not merely hours. It doesn't mean after the interval training you don't do anything else for two or three days, but it does mean you don't do another interval session. You would instead do some aerobic running or cross-training.

However, if you are doing interval training, it takes more out of you and stresses your central nervous system, too, so full recovery can take 48 to 72 hours or longer. Interval work is done leading up to races. We work "slow to fast" to prevent injury. If you work out of order and put a lot of interval training in your base phase when you should be upping your mileage (volume), you are working against your goals, and your chances of injuries increase significantly.

Applying the Long-Term Plan

I'll bet you're asking yourself, "How do I apply all this information I've read to my own situation and training?" In this section, I will work through a sample plan and direct you on which type of workouts fit each phase. You'll see how to turn these ideas into an injury-free training program for yourself.

Let's say your New Year's resolution is to get in shape and lose a few pounds over the next couple of months. You even feel motivated to run a few races over the summer, with the big goal of setting a PR in your local 10k race in the middle of August. So you have roughly 220 to 225 days to get in shape and prepare for these races culminating with this big event. (Don't stress out if you have a little less time; the concepts are the same regardless of how many days you have.)

Now we need to plan what you are going to do (and when, where, and why) during your different phases. You will need to spend 50 percent of your total time doing general types of running and conditioning (easy road running, or base miles), calisthenics (push-ups, pull-ups, and so on), and weight training. Then you should allot the next 25 percent of time to specific preparation (preseason workouts, anaerobic threshold runs, and so on). The next 20 percent of your time will be spent in your competitive phase, and the final 5 percent will be spent on the peaking period.

Aerobic running is easy running where your heart rate stays between 120 and 160 bpm. Anaerobic running is harder running (speed work, intervals, etc.) where your heart rate will be 170+ bpm. Training is a combination of both types of runs. It is the balance between the two types of running that is most important. You should incorporate both into your workouts and not get stuck in one mode too much.

Starting at the End

When you are planning your schedule, I find that it is much easier to start with your ending date and work toward the beginning of your season. I have heard many coaches and athletes regretting that they or their team peaked too early or too late. This is a very easy problem to correct if you just spend a little time planning and adjusting your time-line to peak at the right time.

Okay, back to the 220 days we have to work with on your plan. Let's begin by looking at how much time you will need in the peaking phase first. You will need to spend 5 percent of your total time in the peaking period. Let's round this to 14 days, as I prefer to deal with full weeks of training (remember the 7-day microcycles). I now know that I will be spending the last two weeks of this total time period doing peaking workouts and reducing volume, to allow me to peak at the right time.

The next time period will be the 20 percent allotted to the higher-intensity phase or the competitive season. This percentage equals 44 days, which I will again round to 42 days, or six full weeks that you will spend focused on the competitive phase of training, preceding the two-week peaking period.

Immediately preceding the competitive phase will be a 25 percent period of specific training. This will amount to 55 days or about eight full weeks. During this phase, the emphasis will be on making the transition from base training to preparing to do more specific work to get ready for the competitive season.

Finally—or "beginningly"—you will spend the first 50 percent of your total time (110 days) on base training and general fitness. Actually, the number of days you have left for your beginning phase is 108 days, because of rounding up and down. But that's okay—we've kept the time emphasis focused where it needs to be: on reaching your peak when you want to.

Here's How You'll Run It

So your training program will go something like this (actual days may be slightly more or less due to rounding):

Phase	Weeks	Percent of Total Time
Base	15 weeks	50 percent
Specific training	8 weeks	25 percent
Competitive	6 weeks	20 percent
Peaking	2 weeks	5 percent

This simple division of time periods will allow you to prioritize different aspects of your training, reminding yourself of what is important during each time period. I typically plan and write workouts for an entire season for each of our distance groups before their summer training begins. Certainly there are times when I adjust a workout or a series of workouts depending on how my athletes are adapting to the stress loads, but this initial plan gives me a guideline and focus to the running I will have my athletes do.

The "Write" Way to Train Smart

All of this leads to the importance of keeping a training journal or diary. You want to keep track of what you've done and how you feel during certain time ranges and intensities. Seeing your gradual but steady progress will also remind you that this is a process that takes time and will help keep you from being too greedy.

It's important to write down the focus of your training during each segment so you can check whether, as a highly motivated athlete, you're training too much. Reviewing your training will tell you that, if you need to work on speed, then you need to reduce the volume. Motivated runners doing too much volume during the intensity phase are counter-productive to their goal.

If you don't want to write down all your workouts for an entire season, that's quite alright. But I do suggest you at least write down on a calendar what phase of training you're in and the focus of that phase. This information will help you determine the volume and percentages of intensity you should be running throughout your overall plan. This will also help you plan progressive workouts and avoid skipping steps. Skipping steps and progressing too quickly through volume and/or intensity levels are the biggest culprits that lead to injuries or illness.

Volume or Base Training Period

Now let's get started. Running for volume or building a base is the first step in getting to your goal injury-free. During your first few weeks of training, pay careful attention to the messages your body is sending. You can definitely expect to have some soreness and fatigue, as it will take a full month to adapt.

Now that we have established time periods and focus of training, it's time to talk more about how to build volume in your running. You should start at 40 to 55 percent of your volume goal, then add 7 to 10 percent volume increases each week until you reach 100 percent volume. This process should take no less than four to five weeks and no more than seven to eight weeks, and then you will maintain 90 to 100 percent volume for the rest of the base period. I will usually have my athletes build to 100 percent volume over a five- to six-week period.

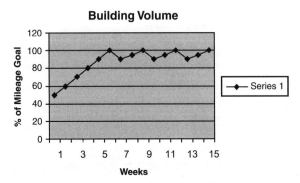

Volume building graph.

So if my goal mileage for this year is 50 miles a week, and I plan to run 25 miles the first week of training, then I begin adding 4 to 5 miles per week to my workout schedule. This process will have you running at full volume in five to six weeks. If you are a more experienced runner coming back after a relative short layoff, then a three- to five-week build-up will probably work best for you. If you are a beginning runner, you may want to start at a lower volume and take a full six to eight weeks to build up to 100 percent.

Once your base building period is complete, you've still got about half of your 15-week base phase to maintain and strengthen your base through continued high-volume training. If your volume goal is 60 miles per week, then in the second half of your base training phase you should run between 54 and 60 miles per week.

Remember during this period to undulate your miles. When you undulate your miles, you take a few steps forward and one backward with your volume. This slight step back is a key for more complete adaptation. So you run 54 (90 percent) one week, then 57, then 60. This variation allows the body to recover and rest and aids in your adaptation process. Even though the miles may vary, you are still building a strong aerobic base that will get you fit and keep you healthy and—most important—prepare you for the next phase of your training program.

You will need to compliment your base running (lots of miles), with some strength and speed work. These two components will not be the focus of your training, but you still need to keep your muscles activated and not forget speed and strength in your volume running. Two good examples of strength and speed training are hills and strides.

We run hills or mountains about once a week for about 12 to 15 percent of our base training mileage. If you are training at 60 miles per week, then you would need to run around 7 to 9 miles each week on a hilly or mountainous course. You also will need to understand how different topography will impact your training program. You may live in a very hilly environment and not have to dedicate a special workout to hill training; instead, you may need to seek out flat areas for your low-intensity workouts.

Strides or accelerations are the most common choice for keeping in touch with our faster twitch muscles during the base phase. Strides are a series of short fast runs, generally about 100 yards at a fast pace, repeated 8 to 10 times.

Our muscles are made up of two types of fibers, slow twitch and fast twitch. If you don't work your fast twitch (slow twitch are regularly used), they'll go dormant; and when you try to move faster, it won't happen. By doing strides at the end of run, you awaken your fast-twitch fibers and have them active and ready when you want to move faster.

Most often we accomplish this by ending our easy workouts with six to eight 100-meter strides on the grass. These strides are normally run at an 800- to 1,500-meter race pace or faster. This type of training utilizes fast-twitch fibers and doesn't allow them to become too dormant during the base phase. This will help by gradually using and building these muscle fibers into their racing shape.

I believe you'll see big benefits if you incorporate both of these elements into your training. It will give you the variety in your training and depth in your fitness that assists you in becoming a stronger, faster, and healthier athlete.

Another key weekly run during this phase is the long run. One day each week you should complete a long, easy run that makes up around 20 percent of your total week's mileage. If you're running 60 miles per week, then this long run should be 12 miles. I generally tell runners to do this workout on the weekend, early in the morning. This allows more time for rest and recovery than the traditional midweek workout. Although this workout is of relatively low intensity, the mere length of it takes a toll on how your body feels and responds.

Specific Training

In the next phase of training, the pre-competitive phase, you complete the base phase and transition into more specialized training. During this phase, your mileage is still relatively high and you will begin running a few of your workouts a little faster. You are gradually preparing your body to tolerate faster running as your intensity is still increasing methodically. This particular stage is critical in injury prevention. If this phase of running is not done properly, you will most definitely have problems adapting to the increased intensities of the next phase.

A typical week would include a long run, an anaerobic threshold run, a hill or mountain run, and a moderate road run of 5 to 6 miles at 160 bpm heart rate. The remaining days are recovery runs, or you might even take one or two of these days off. You should also continue your strides following your easy runs two or three times a week.

You'll begin to see that each phase prepares you to transition into the next phase, which lessens your risk of injury and illness. Many times injuries and illness will occur as a result of changing volume or intensities too quickly. Making progress through each phase and being prepared for the next one will eliminate most of these risk factors.

Competitive Phase

Just like all phases of training, the competitive phase has a primary focus, which is to sharpen and prepare the body to run faster. Running fast is a risk factor in itself; while running fast, your body will absorb more impact with each running stride. You will need to pay attention to the quality of your running, as the volume of your running is not the primary focus anymore. You may begin to cut some mileage from your program as the competitive season wears on, depending on your experience and the racing distances you have planned, and this section will help you determine how much to cut back and when.

During this phase, you will spend some time developing tactics and making psychological preparations. These factors will be important during the competitive phase. These factors sometimes are neglected until the peaking period, but it is important to begin developing them throughout the competitive season. You can refine what works best for you during the peaking phase.

Even if you're not preparing to compete in a race, you still need to go through this competitive phase, but you can just call it a combination phase. It involves sharpening some different muscles and preparing your body to train in a different way. This new stage is an essential part of your development as a runner and is needed to keep you injury-free and sharp. You improve your body and your mind in stages; this is part of the entire training cycle.

Peaking Phase

You can end up rushing the peaking phase if you did not have good progress or development during the competitive period. Like all phases, the peaking phase has its own focus, and it's a time to allow your body to fully acclimate to any stresses you have by severely cutting back volume. You may increase intensity here, but be cautious about the volume of hard work during this time. This should allow you to continue to sharpen up. This procedure will prepare you to run your fastest times of the year.

By this point in your training cycle, you should have experimented with different race tactics and strategies and decided on what will work best for you in your final couple of races. You have made it this far without injury or illness; don't risk overdoing it now. If you've spent much time around coaches during the peaking phase, then I'm sure you have heard the saying, "The hay's in the barn." This means the work should already be done, and too many things can go wrong by trying to get any extra work during this phase. Rest and recovery will serve you best now.

This doesn't mean you discontinue running altogether. However, you need to reduce your volume to 50 to 60 percent of your previous levels and pick, choose, and plan where and when to work hard, and follow it up with more R & R. All that's left is for you to put out that great effort at the end, set that new personal record, and stay injury-free.

Intensity, Volume, and Their Relationship

As you begin your base phase and build mileage gradually, intensity should not be your primary focus, but you should still allow one or two days a week when you are running at 70 to 75 percent effort. Most of your base training will be going out for easy runs or running for strength, all of which should at least be done at 60 percent of your maximum heart rate or greater. Scientists have concluded that if you don't work out at 60 percent of your heart's capability, you won't increase your capacity.

As your base training progresses and you are nearing the specific period of training, you can begin running one or two workouts per week at 70 to 80 percent intensity. Then, near the end of your specific training period, you will begin transitioning into the competitive season. At this point, you can begin running intervals and other workouts at 82 to 85 percent intensity. From this point, I suggest only increasing your intensity level by 3 to 4 percent. Larger increases will lead to erratic performances and increase your risk of injury. Remember to change the intensity of your workouts every 21 to 28 days, as this will help you to continue improving.

As the competitive season rolls around, you may want to reduce your volume by 5 percent, and reduce it by another 5 percent toward the middle of your season. As you reduce volume, your legs will eventually begin to feel more rested, which will improve the quality of your workouts. Over the last few weeks of your competitive season and the two weeks of your peaking phase, you will want to reduce volume gradually down to 50 or 60 percent of your high mileage point.

During this time, you should have some very high-quality workouts. But when you're feeling fresher, be careful not to overdo it on your hard days. Don't waste your best performances in workouts—your special efforts should be saved for your biggest races. It is also important to be very careful when your volume and intensity are both at high points (in the high 80 percent range), because that's when you are most susceptible to injury.

This period usually occurs over the last few weeks of the competitive period. If you overtrain during this phase, you may come down with a cold or, worse, a season-ending injury. This is the time to be most in tune with how your body is feeling and adapting to the volume and intensity that you are running.

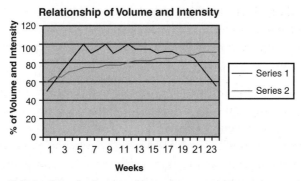

Relationship of volume and intensity.

In the preceding chart, series 1 represents volume (or mileage) and series 2 represents intensity. Notice that as your mileage and intensity lines cross, you are nearing the end of your competitive phase and beginning your peaking period.

The point where mileage volume and intensity meet is one of the most vulnerable for illness and injury. Your body is at a high stress point, and any dip in your rest or recovery may result in something negative. Doing everything right at this critical time will pay off, keeping you healthy and allowing you to fully benefit from the peaking phase that comes next.

The Law of Reversibility

There will be times when you need to take an extended break, whether it is for injuries, illness, or just a vacation from running. The one question I am frequently asked is, "How long does it take to get out of shape?"

If you take a full two weeks off from running, you may have a slight decline in your fitness, but you can regain this fitness over the first three to four weeks of running again. If you take a longer break from running, say six to eight weeks, and you are a relative newcomer to running, you may lose 40 to 50 percent of your current fitness. If you've been running for a number of years, you won't lose as much fitness as the newcomer.

If you can do a couple of quality sessions during your break (I know— that doesn't really sound like a break), maybe run twice a week for two weeks, then your loss of fitness will be very minimal. Even though you may lose some fitness, it is important that you take scheduled breaks at the end of your competitive seasons. These much-needed breaks allow you to recharge your batteries by replenishing vitamins, minerals, and your soul.

The Law of Specificity

Mozart didn't become a great musician by running down the road; he did it by playing the piano many hours per day. The SAID principle stands for *Specific Adaptation Imposed Demand* and basically means that you must run in order to improve as a runner. Got that? Okay, it's a little more specific than that: it means your body will adapt exactly to the types of running you will be doing.

When I first began coaching, I probably coached a lot of the middle-distance and distance runners the same. (Not probably—I did.) Needless to say, the middle-distance runners didn't perform as well as I would have liked. Over the first few years, we didn't have a national champion in the 800- or 1500- meter races. I'm sure you've heard that knowledge is power, and as I learned more and changed the workouts for the middle-distance runners, their performances began to soar.

The main adjustment I made was to train this group more specifically for their events. This entailed doing more training in the weight room and more track workouts. I'm not suggesting this type of training is what's best for you, but it does show that making your training more specific can elicit a much better result. Since changing our middle-distance workouts to be more specific, we have won 22 individual national titles in the 800- and 1500-meter races alone.

If you are training for lifelong fitness and you have no desire to race, then you should run enough to have a healthy heart, muscles, and mind. If you are going to race a marathon, then your training should be more volume oriented than training for a 5k. Not training for your race distance puts you at greater risk of injury during the actual event.

The Least You Need to Know

◆ Periodization ties all aspects of a program together.

◆ The base phase will determine what goals you reach in your running program.

◆ When you are injured, you will not be able to pick right up where you left off, so take your time.

◆ Doing things the right way takes some thought and time, but it's well worth it to keep you injury-free.

Chapter 4

Increasing Your Running Energy

In This Chapter

- Why you should run longer, not faster
- How to work at your best heart rate
- What kind of energy your body uses as fuel
- How the heart grows with your running program

Energy—we all need more of it. In fact, a lot of people complain that they don't have nearly enough. This chapter is somewhat technical, but I assure you that when you learn how these systems function, you will have a leg up on staying injury-free.

The energy you expend while running can be broken into two types: aerobic and anaerobic. Energy burned aerobically means that it is broken down in the presence of oxygen. Energy broken down anaerobically is energy without the presence of oxygen. Running almost always involves a combination of the two.

What Drives Your Engine?

As you run aerobically, you will be running at easier paces. The oxygen you are inhaling will pass through your lungs and be processed in your red blood cells. Breaking down energy with the help of oxygen will prevent the accumulation of lactic acid and other by-products that eventually slow you down.

The converse of this would be breaking down energy anaerobically, or without the presence of oxygen. As you run faster and the demands of running require more energy, your lungs cannot supply enough oxygen for the breakdown of energy. This produces by-products such as lactic acid and hydrogen ions, which eventually accumulate and will negatively affect your efforts.

Lactic acid is often misunderstood. Lactic acid is what causes that burning sensation in your muscles when you run fast. We all build some lactic acid as we do low levels of exercise; as the intensity goes up and our heart rate rises, we produce more. At the point that your body can't remove it as fast as you produce it, it's a negative. But when the body is trained correctly, lactic acid can be your friend and become an energy source!

Hydrogen ions are the waste elements produced during anaerobic running. They attach themselves to your muscles as you exercise. That causes the tightness that you can feel as you run faster. In racing circles, this is sometimes called "locking up" or "the bear jumped on your back." Everyone who races has either seen it or felt it. Now you know what causes it.

It is also important for you to understand the fuels your body uses for energy, primarily glycogen and fats. Glycogen is a fancy name for carbohydrates that we have stored for later use. Fats are also stored—and hopefully we'll burn them away as well! Understanding the basics of how these fuels are processed with and without oxygen will give you a better idea of how to plan your workouts.

Building Your Base

Understanding the basic principles of aerobic and anaerobic running will help keep you from exceeding your optimal intensities and speeds while base training. You need to build a base before going on to more advanced training. You should avoid overdoing it, commonly known as overtraining.

As you run at lower intensity levels and heart rates (less than 160 bpm), your runs are much more aerobic in nature. When training aerobically, you will be able to run for longer periods without producing large accumulations of lactic acid or hydrogen ions. This type of training includes long endurance runs, recovery runs, aerobic threshold running, or any training at a level where you're working at a rate that allows you to process enough oxygen for energy breakdown.

Watch Your Step

If you're running too fast, you might be working against your goal of dropping weight and cutting time. Depending on how your body adapts and recovers from your training workouts, you can proceed faster or slower with your training.

There is a fine line that determines whether a run is more aerobic or anaerobic. Individuals vary, but this fine line is somewhere around 165 to 175 heartbeats per minute. As you run at higher heart rates (greater than 175 bpm), your breakdown of energy becomes more anaerobic.

All running (races and practices) have aerobic or anaerobic breakdown of energy and use combinations of both throughout the run. For example, a marathoner who runs for a long period of time is probably running 98 percent aerobic and 2 percent anaerobic. At the other end of the spectrum, someone training for a 100-meter race might be training 98 percent anaerobic and 2 percent aerobic.

Anaerobic training can be a very beneficial workout as you're trying to improve your times. When doing this type of training, be sure to warm up and cool down properly, as anaerobic training requires greater muscular output and will leave metabolic waste that needs to be removed at the end of the workout. The benefits of anaerobic training include greater efficiency and improved muscular output and performance.

Distance	Aerobic/anaerobic
Marathon	98%/2%
Half marathon	94%/6%
10k	90%/10%
5k	80%/20%
100m	2%/98%

Certainly the longer and easier the run, the more energy you're burning aerobically. The caloric expenditure of a highly trained person can be between 1,000 and 1,200 calories in a particular workout, whereas a beginning athlete might only burn 300 to 500 calories in a workout.

Understanding these factors is very important in your training, whether you're a novice or an experienced athlete.

It's All About Heart (Rate)

When working at anaerobic fitness or running, you need to be careful, because you are running at a faster pace. To run at this level, your body will have to be completely warmed up and ready to go, as the workout will be more strenuous on your muscles, bones, tendons, and joints.

Anaerobic threshold training is an important part of being able to race up to your potential. We work on training this energy system quite extensively. It is important that this type of training be done progressively, going from slower paces to faster ones. In order to improve significantly without injury and receive the biggest bang for your buck, you must run just under or right up to your anaerobic threshold level. Remember, the anaerobic threshold is that fine line between 165 to 175 bpm heart rate, where the utilization of energy is approximately 50 percent aerobic and 50 percent anaerobic.

Road Blocks

It is very important to do an adequate cooldown; this will ensure the removal of metabolic waste that accumulates during this type of training. You can find more on this in Chapter 6.

Young runners often want to run faster because they can, but this will not yield the results they desire. The object is to run in this specific heart rate range, and eventually you'll be able to run faster and faster *yet stay at the same heart rate* and thus not accumulate lactic acid as time goes on and adaptation occurs. An example of this would be for you to run at 170 heart rate; let's say that ended up being an eight–minute-mile pace. You should repeat this type of running once every 7 to 14 days over a two- to four-week period. Eventually you will be running a 7:45- to 7:50-minute mile at the 170 bpm target heart rate.

We try to work right around the anaerobic threshold level (168 to 172 bpm heart rate). We'll do medium to long runs (4 to 10 miles) at this heart rate, right under the anaerobic level, so you're removing lactic acid and hydrogen ions a little faster than you're accumulating them. Therefore you can still run fast, and for long periods, without accumulating large amounts of lactic acid and hydrogen ions. This type of training will provide tremendous improvement for your investment.

Taking your heart rate (either manually or with a monitor) is the best way to know when you're at or just under this threshold. When we're on training runs, I have the runners stop and take each other's heart rate for 10 seconds. Multiply that number by 6 and you have your heart rate for a full minute. You want to do it that way because, if you try to take it for a full minute, your heart rate will continue to decline and not be representative of your workout rate.

Runner Facts

You can never take your heart rate too often. Knowing the number of beats your heart is producing per minute tells you what "zone" you are working in.

VO2 Max—It Means Better, Longer, Faster Running

What is VO2 Max? The textbook answer is, "It's the total amount of oxygen you can inspire (the amount of oxygen you can breathe into your lungs) per minute of exercise, divided by your kilograms of body weight." An easier way to think about this is, it's the amount of oxygen your body can put to good use. A description that I often use is that it's like a car—the larger the gas tank, the farther and faster the car can go; the less the car weighs, the longer it can travel. Your lungs are the gas tank and your body weight is the car size. I probably don't have to say that you'll have the best chance of success with a big gas tank and a light frame.

Increased VO2 Max can have a dramatic effect on your performance. In the 1500-meter run, for example, it could be as much as 7 seconds improvement per 2 milliliters for an elite runner and as much as 12 to 15 seconds improvement for a beginner. Over the longer races, it improves even more. So in a 10k race, this could be 40 seconds to a minute for a 2 milliliter VO2 Max increase for the elite, and 90 seconds to 2 minutes for the beginner. As you increase your VO2 Max, it increases your chances of running faster.

Female athletes have a little lower VO2 Max for several reasons. One, they have a little less lean body mass and a little more fat than male runners do, to insulate and protect their female reproductive organs. Elite males can have 3 to 5 percent body fat; elite females may have two or three times that amount and be considered just as fit. The higher lean body mass in males allows them to develop a little higher VO2 Max than females. Other contributing factors to reaching a higher VO2 Max are just time and age. The more you work at developing aerobic fitness and the more volume (miles) you are able to run will certainly increase your lung capacity and give you higher VO2 Max values.

"Running economy" is another term we use frequently. Being able to utilize a large amount of VO2 Max without going into an anaerobic state is very important. Highly trained athletes are able to use 80 to 85 percent of their VO2 Max without going into an anaerobic effort. Say they have a VO2 Max of 80, and they can work at 80 percent of that; they can operate at 64 VO2 Max without breaking down any energy source without the presence of oxygen. So increasing your running economy by running faster and faster without going into an anaerobic effort is key to sustaining fast running.

The Power of a Big Heart

One of your basic goals of beginning a program should be to increase cardiac output. An added benefit will be that you will increase the strength and size of your heart. This is important because you'll be able to pump more blood per contraction of your heart. This is called "stroke volume," which is very important for a developing runner. If you can pump more blood per contraction, your heart gets stronger and its maximum amount of beats per minute improves. The larger and stronger your heart becomes, the more it increases the stroke volume. You can increase your heart size to as large as 50 percent more than a normal heart, which allows you to pump that much more blood.

Taking care of your heart and lungs aids you in fitness and injury prevention—not just typical aches and pains, but overall conditioning. When your heart pumps more blood, your muscles and tissues will be able to get more oxygen. The volume of the blood that you have in your body will increase. This results in an increase in the number of red blood cells. Therefore the system will work much more efficiently and effectively.

Lung tissue can also be increased as much as twofold. Your ability to process and have more oxygen readily available will improve as the size of lung tissue increases. This will make the system more effective. As you bring more oxygen to your blood cells, your muscles can do more work. All of this keeps you healthier and running fast!

It All Starts with a Good Base

Aerobic training is the primary type of training you will be doing during your "base training" phase. This is what we do in our off season more so than in the competitive phase—in the competitive phase, we run aerobically mainly as recovery runs, easy runs, and long runs.

It is very important that your base be as complete as possible during the off season—this will have a profound effect on your peaking process when you gear up for big competitions. So the better your base, the higher your potential.

Slow Twitch and Fast Twitch: The Long and Short of It

Muscle tissue is another way of measuring success and potential of athletes. Muscle cells are made up of fast-twitch and slow-twitch fibers. Endurance runners have a predominance of slow-twitch fibers, middle-distance runners have a combination of both, and sprinters have a high amount of fast-twitch fibers. These ratios of fast- and slow-twitch fibers are good indicators of potential in certain events. A genetic component comes into play in assessing your potential for specific distances or sprints. If you have more slow-twitch fibers, you'll have a greater potential to develop for longer distances.

Very sophisticated lab tests can tell you if you have slow- or fast-twitch fibers, but regular folks can just consider the following: if you are able to "kick into another gear" as the race ends, or if you can sprint faster than most of your workout partners, then you probably have a higher percentage of fast-twitch fibers than your fellow runners.

Although runners are born with a certain amount of fast- and slow-twitch fibers, these fibers are actually very trainable. Take a distance runner with 65 percent fast-twitch fibers and only 35 percent slow-twitch fibers; through training, you can increase the size of the slow-twitch fibers and decrease the size of the fast-twitch fibers. Even though the ratio of fibers is 65/35 in number, it's not uncommon that these fibers could end up being more like 50/50 in total size during the base phase of training while working only aerobically and doing a high volume of training.

Cells Incarcerate Energy

Every cell needs energy. Inside the cell is a peanut-shaped component called the *mitochondria*, which is the powerhouse of the cell that helps us break down energy in the form of glycogen and fats.

Glycogen is carbohydrates that we have stored in our liver and muscle cells. Athletes break down varying amounts of glycogen and fat in their workouts. A high-level endurance athlete can store 1,500 to 1,900 kilocalories of glycogen, enough energy to sustain a two-hour, high-intensity workout. As you work harder, you will get most of your energy from glycogen, but you will still get some energy from fat.

Runner Facts

It takes twice the amount of energy to break down 1 gram of fat as it does to break down 1 gram of carbohydrate.

Fat is the primary energy source when we are working out easier and at lower intensity. If you are trying to lose weight, it is smart to pay special attention to your heart rate. This will help you burn more fat. If you're just starting out and wanting to lose a few pounds, it's wise to keep a lower heart rate, somewhere between 130 to 155 bpm.

So here's a warning: when you exercise too hard and too fast and think you are going to burn fat, it won't work. Your heart rate is going to be so high that your primary source of energy will be mostly glycogen, not fat. In other words, you'll burn a lot more fat with longer periods of exercise at a lower heart rate. This will also aid your fitness level and help you prevent injury.

A Shift in Running Theory

The long slow distance (LSD) training of the 1970s—just miles upon miles only—was great for fitness but led to poor performances. The running movement of the time overemphasized this type of running, and higher-intensity running (tempo runs, intervals, repetition running) was not emphasized, leading to poor performances. Distance running is a great way to build a base, but you should include faster running in your training as you finish your base work and move into precompetitive and competitive seasons.

Aerobic running can be done for long periods of time, an hour to two hours. This running should not be exhaustive, where it's done for a long period of time at a high intensity; it should be done at lower heart rates (130 to 150 bpm) and lower energy rates. This will lesson the demands of quick, high-energy utilization and also reduce oxygen demands. The duration of these aerobic runs will aid in increasing your VO2 Max.

There are several drawbacks to only doing this type of training. Because aerobic running heart rates are lower, this does not emphasize economy of running at faster paces. In other words, aerobic running teaches the body to use energy over a long period of time and to increase VO2 Max, not to prepare the body for racing fast. But remember that aerobic running is a very important step in preparing to eventually race fast.

Cranking It Up a Gear, but Not into Overdrive

The next type of running you should incorporate into your program is fast-distance/tempo running—many times we call this anaerobic-threshold running. These runs can vary from 4 to 10 miles. Don't forget to include your proper warm-up and cooldown by easy jogging for 10 to 15 minutes. This will help remove metabolic waste and relax tight muscles. This type of running places a higher demand on the cardio-vascular system, the circulatory and energy system. The primary benefit of this type of training is it allows you to run much closer to racing paces without any large accumulations of lactic acid.

Most runners use this kind of running in their training program. I believe anaerobic-threshold running is the "big money" when you are looking for significant improvements at racing 5k to marathon distances. You will get more benefit out of this kind of training than any other for the time spent doing it, yet it's not as difficult and stressful on the muscles and bones as other types of running. This will allow you to stay healthy. As you go harder into interval training or repetition training, it puts a higher amount of stress on the muscles and bones, which can lead to injury.

Interval running can be a very effective tool in helping you run faster. It's very important to understand this type of training before you head out the door. Before running intervals, it is imperative that you've had a thorough warm-up. When you're warmed up properly, you're less at risk of injuring muscles or tendons with strains or pulls. (We cover warming up and cooling down in Chapter 6.)

Interval Example Program

Weeks 1–3: Interval running 15×400 m @ 82% intensity

Weeks 4–6: Interval running 12×400 m @ 85% intensity

Weeks 7–9: Interval running 10×400 m @ 88% intensity

Week 10: Interval running 9×400 m @ 90% intensity

Week 11: Interval running 7×400 m @ 91% intensity

Week 12: Interval running 6×400 m @ 92% intensity

Intensity is the percentage of your best time at a given distance. If your best 400 meters is 70 seconds, then 82 percent intensity means you will need to do the interval workout at 83 seconds per 400 m.

Interval running consists of faster running timed over distances. Distances can range from 200 meters, 400 meters to 1600-meter or 3000-meter repeats. The total volume of these intervals will be directly related to the speed of each one run.

If you're a beginning runner, you may want to do 10×400 meters as a workout. The intensity at which we do these will have a direct impact on the amount of rest and recovery you need to take between each interval. As you run each repetition, the interval of active rest needs to be administered accordingly. When doing an interval workout, use a running watch as your guide. Start the watch when you begin the interval, then hit the stop button as you cross the line. Begin the rest period by clicking again and measuring the rest period.

Intensity is the key factor when working at interval training. When working at lower intensities, such as 70 percent intensity, the recovery is very short and the volume of total interval work can be higher (maybe 15 or 20×400-meter repeats). But when doing intervals at 90 percent intensity and higher, the recovery is going to be longer and the total volume of work much smaller.

Novice runners sometimes shy away from interval training because they are inexperienced and feel it's not valuable to them. But I believe interval training, when done properly, is applicable to most runners of all ages. Interval training can be adjusted to the level of any runner of any ability level. At the same time, one should take caution not to overdo any particular session (too much volume or running at too high an intensity for fitness level). Intervals need to be introduced slowly into your program and need to be progressive in their usage.

I typically use this type of training for 10 to 12 weeks. When we first begin our interval running, our intensity level is around 82 to 83 percent effort. Every three weeks I will increase this percentage by 3 to 4 percent. As the percentages get higher, the total volume of work will decrease.

Fartlek: It's Not What It Sounds Like

Fartlek, a Swedish term, means "speed play," as we start to go from off-season training to in-season training. This can be done on a dirt road or through the forest. It's not as structured as interval training. You can be as creative as your imagination or have some basic structure. You may have a goal of running certain times or various distances, or you may sometimes just run how you feel. Recoveries can also be as structured or unstructured as you like. It's not as organized, but it can be an important part of your training regimen as you get a little mentally stressed or burned out. This is will allow you to have a good, hard training session without the stress of having to meet a certain time or distance.

You'll use all these types of training in varying degrees at different times of the year. As you do your base training, you will be running more aerobically; as you get into shape or get into the competitive season, you'll use more interval training.

A lot of it depends on your distance goals. If you're training to run a 1-mile race or seeking a best time, you will need to do more interval training. But if you're training for a 10k or a marathon, you'll do less interval training. Set goals and follow the proper kind of training for them. This will provide direction for your running and allow you to avoid injuries.

One new concept is multitiered training, which is training for several different racing distances over a one- or two-week plan. Many runners tend to stagnate in their training, as they do not work at varying paces. Multitiered training allows you to emphasize different kinds of training as you work toward a race or try to reach your goals. So you might do all of these kinds of training over a 14-day period, and the emphasis will shift depending on what you need the most.

Beware of Overtraining

Overtraining is an important consideration when trying to stay injury-free. When your motivation is high, so is your danger of overtraining. You need to monitor this no matter what phase you are in. One way is to take a basal heart rate every morning. First thing in the morning, before you get out of bed, find your carotid artery with your index and middle fingers. Count the amount of beats that your heart is pumping per minute.

Start with 0 on the first beat, 1 on the second beat, 2 on the third, and so on for the full minute. Don't start with 1, as you want to count as if the heart is just filling up with blood on the first contraction. Take your heart rate over a few mornings and average it to establish a benchmark as your basal metabolic rate.

If your heart rate increases by 10 to 15 percent over a couple of mornings, it can be an indication of overtraining. When this happens, back off your training immediately; this will help you avoid injury or sickness. Many times this is the only signal that you are overtrained. It can come from running too much or too hard. It can also come from improper nutrition or a lack of rest and sleep.

High Intensity: A Quick Route to Injuries

There's a time and place for all types of running. You should only get into high-intensity training once you have a sufficient base. Significant research in training younger athletes with high-intensity running shows that it's not very productive; overdoing it can burn you out and lead to injuries. Training with long, steady, lower-intensity programs seems to be a lot more helpful in long-term development and progress.

Third-world countries like Kenya and Ethiopia have many world-class runners who actually weren't trained to run per se. They ran to and from school, or while doing chores, and so on. Many long, steady runs helped develop their aerobic systems and their muscle and tendon strength in their legs over long periods, without high intensity as the primary focus. Developing their cardiovascular systems with less stress has led to astounding results. This foundation provides a great base to pull upon for higher-intensity running later.

You can benefit from this research by applying these principles to your training plan. Build your strength with long, steady runs. Take your time and enjoy your experience as you meander along; it will be healthy and build your base, thus preventing injury.

The Least You Need to Know

◆ Find a program that works for you and your body and lifestyle.

◆ Don't overtrain, even on your best days.

◆ Time to relax is important—physically and mentally.

Part 2

Finding Your Stride

Running helps you develop a healthy lifestyle, and part of that is finding the right weight. There is a right way and wrong way to manage your weight, and a few extra pounds shouldn't keep you from reaching your goals—in running or in life. First we'll talk about getting the right food to fuel your engine.

The most important yet underrated and overlooked parts of running may be the warm-up and the cooldown. We'll look at why that is and why they're both necessary, then get into detail on putting stretching and strength training to work for you.

We'll wrap up this part with something we all love but never think we have enough time for: sleep. One of the many myths about training is that more is always better. But it's not. Over-training is a first step, and then a leap, in the wrong direction, and it starts with not getting enough R & R: Rest and Recovery.

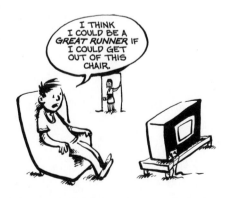

Chapter 5

Nutrition and Body Weight

In This Chapter

- ◆ Why eating smart prevents injuries
- ◆ What fuel is best to keep you from breaking down
- ◆ What foods give you the best chance to stay healthy
- ◆ Understanding your body type to stay healthy
- ◆ Smart weight-loss goals to avoid injury

Approximately 60 percent of all Americans are overweight (men, 18–24 percent body fat; women, 25–29 percent body fat) or obese (men, 25 percent or more body fat; women, 30 percent or more body fat), and these percentages are increasing every year. Is the solution to this problem exercise, better nutrition, or both?

I hope this chapter will help you determine how using running and nutrition can get you to your recommended or ideal body weight (men, 6–17 percent body fat; women, 10–24 percent body fat).

Making Smart Eating Choices

Some recreational runners tend to eat larger meals than they should to maintain or lose body weight. They think that because they run they can eat as much as they want! However, these same runners will gain unnecessary weight over the course of several months or a year. The weight gain is not that noticeable at first, but it does eventually add up. This can affect even those runners who run as much as 45 miles a week. They can underestimate how much they're eating by as much as 15 to 30 percent.

We can be confused about how many calories we burn in a given day. Difficulties in planning our daily meals can thwart our efforts to lose those extra pounds or maintain our ideal weight. Having said that, losing weight can be easier—you just need to consume fewer calories than you burn. With some basic knowledge, you can accurately count the number of calories you eat and use daily.

The biggest challenge will be identifying portion size in the different food groups and how many portions you should eat per day. Restaurants will typically serve double and triple portions per entrée. This problem is exacerbated because we almost always eat everything on our plates, even when this leads to overeating.

What to Eat, What Not to Eat

We tend to think the size of our bowl or plate is the amount of food we should eat. If you don't think in terms of standard portions, it's hard to estimate how many calories you're consuming. Guessing how many calories you're eating isn't reliable: we tend to be "optimistic" when we're eating larger meals. Therefore it's important to know portions of food and calories per portion if we are to maintain or lose weight.

No two people will have the exact same problems (basal metabolism rate, genetics, eating habits, workout routines, and so on) in reaching their goal weights. If you're more worried about your health than your weight, you can indeed be better off being fat and fit rather than lean and unfit. We often focus too much on weight, which diminishes the importance of fitness. We should focus on the health benefits that come with simply being more active. If you become fitter and leaner through your training and nutritional program, no matter what your starting weight is, you will become a more efficient runner.

Runner Facts _____

Most athletes trying to lose weight immediately start cutting back on their fat intake. Instead of just cutting out nonessential fats, they also cut out healthy fats, including nuts and olives. Some types of fat help slow digestion and provide a sense of fullness. It is important to get 25 percent of your daily calories from good fats by selecting healthy vegetables, nuts, and fish sources.

The runner who is more interested in running fast than getting fit and/or healthy usually wants to know his or her ideal racing weight for 5k to marathon distances. If these athletes lose too much body weight, they can become weak and slow. Many parents and coaches worry about young runners developing anorexia nervosa; this can be a problem among adolescent and college-age female runners. Anorexia affects less than 1 percent of the overall population, but is four to six times more likely in young female runners.

The definition of VO2 Max states that you should divide the amount of oxygen you can inspire per minute of exercise by your kilograms of body weight. This is very significant; a runner would improve about two to three seconds per mile for every pound reduced. This loss of weight will boost VO2 Max, which is essential to increasing distance running potential. The less weight you carry around, the easier it will be to supply more oxygen to your working muscles. Losing a few extra pounds will also make running easier; you will be able to increase your mileage and intensity. So losing weight will help you train harder and stay injury-free.

Runners who want to lose weight to run faster should be sure they are losing fat, not muscle. Fortunately, it is well known that exercise-based weight-loss programs with the aid of good nutrition help you achieve this goal better than only using a fad diet.

How Much Is Enough?

Runners tend to be obsessive/compulsive people who thrive on numbers such as miles run, amount of time run, average pace per mile, and so on. Many runners keep very accurate daily running logs of this information. But many athletes can use help figuring out how many calories they eat and how many they burn during running and cross-training.

If you consume 50 extra calories a day, you would gain 5 pounds in a year. That's one low-calorie sports drink a day. The extra body weight many runners have could simply be the result of drinking to replenish their fluids without paying attention to the caloric intake of the beverage. Drink water!

Watch Your Step

Many times, athletes forget that all calories consumed do count; runners tend to underestimate the amount of calories consumed and overestimate the amount of calories they burn. Runners need to match their nutritional plan to their exercise level.

I suggest a 50/25/25 eating plan, where 50 percent of your calories come from carbohydrates, 25 percent from protein, and 25 percent from fat. With half of your calorie intake coming from carbohydrates, this plan will provide available fuels for your exercise. The rest of your calories will be split evenly between proteins and fats, which will help you feel full longer—this is imperative in losing weight.

When estimating your daily calorie needs for maintaining your current body weight, take your current weight and multiply that by 13. That number will cover your basal metabolism and enough calories for an easy day of activity. So if you weigh 160 pounds, you will need about 2,080 calories per day to maintain your weight at your present activity level. To lose 1 pound each week, you must then create a deficit of 500 calories a day for seven days, as 3,500 calories equals 1 pound.

Then you must make a decision on how you plan to have a deficit of 500 calories per day. The amount of calories you cut from your nutritional program depends a lot on how many calories you're consuming now. If you're only eating 1,500 a day, it seems unreasonable to cut 500 calories a day. But if you're eating 3,500 calories a day, then 500 shouldn't be much of a problem!

Continued weight loss will be a lot easier to manage as you add in your training. Running 1 mile will equal approximately 100 calories of caloric expenditure. If you run 5 miles (500 calorie expenditure) and eat 2,080 calories every day, a 160-pound runner would lose 1 pound per week. Or you can eat 250 fewer calories per day (taking in 1,830 a day) and run 2½ miles per day to come up with the deficit of 500 calories per day. Most experts recommend a loss of no more than 2 pounds per week.

Running every day is the best way to lose weight. If you are not interested or able to do this, running three to five times per week is still a great way to lose weight. Running less often means you'll need to adjust you calorie intake slightly; losing one pound will take about 1½ to 2 weeks.

After you calculate the calories you should be consuming each day to meet your weight-loss goals, you need to decide where you want these calories to come from. If you have determined that your daily caloric goal is 2,080 calories, then 1,040 of those calories should come from carbohydrates, 520 should come from protein, and 520 should come from fat. Not every food you eat will fit into this ratio of carbohydrates, proteins, and fats, but you're trying to get your total daily caloric intake to fall within these ranges.

High-Octane Fuels

Carbohydrates are the body's preferred energy source. Lots of athletes look at the 50 percent carbohydrate recommendation and have a hard time managing to stick to it. They'll think it's not enough, that they need closer to 60 percent or more.

Elite athletes do need a very high percentage of calories from carbohydrates, but recreational runners don't need as many carbohydrates as elite runners. Consuming 50 percent of your daily calories from carbohydrates will provide you with all the energy you need.

Great fruits (approximately 60 calories a portion)
Apple, orange, pear, banana, peach, plum
Canned fruit (in its own juice): ½ cup

Low-starch vegetables (approximately 25 calories a portion)
Carrots, celery, broccoli, green beans: 1 cup raw or ½ cup cooked
Asparagus: 7 cooked, 12–14 raw
Lettuce/raw greens: 1 cup

Vegetables that are high in starch (about 80 calories a portion)

Choose less and use caution!

Beans: ⅓ cup

Corn: ½ cup

Lentils: ½ cup

Baked potato or sweet potato

Pasta and rice (approximately 80 calories a portion)

Couscous: ⅓ cup

Brown or white rice: ⅓ cup

Pasta: ½ cup

Breads/cereal/crackers (approximately 80 calories a portion)

Whole-wheat bread: 1 slice

Pretzels: ¾ oz.

Popcorn (air popped): 3 cups

Rice cakes: 2

Oatmeal: ⅔ cup

You definitely should eat more fruit and vegetables daily. Fruits and vegetables are high in fiber, which causes you to feel full and will help you eat less. Athletes on high-fiber nutritional plans (25–30 grams of fiber per day) tend to eat less fat.

More Fuel for the Fire

Although protein's primary function is to supply energy and rebuild muscle tissue, it also works great for curbing hunger. Protein is best for allowing the stomach to feel full; pound for pound (or in this case ounce for ounce), it satisfies hunger much better than carbohydrates. Eating protein allows you to consume fewer calories but still feel full. This is one good reason why 25 percent of your calories should come from protein.

However, it is important to choose the leanest protein possible. Fats do add flavor to protein but also add calories; you can do without the extra flavor to get rid of the additional calories. Try to limit the number of calories in the protein you choose.

Leanest choices (approximately 35 calories a portion)

Turkey breast: 1 oz.

Chicken breast: 1 oz.

Canned tuna packed in water: 1 oz.

Egg whites: 2 large

Lean choices to consider (approximately 55 calories a portion)

Chicken or turkey (dark meat): 1 oz.

Salmon, trout: 1 oz.

Lean beef (flank steak, top round): 1 oz.

Low-fat luncheon meats: 1 oz.

Dairy products (approximately 90 calories a portion)

Fat-free cottage cheese: 1 cup

Low-fat yogurt: ¾ cup

Low-fat cheese: 2 oz.

Good fats (approximately 50 calories a portion)

Avocado: ⅛

Almonds and cashews: 6

Peanuts: 10

Pistachios: 15

Olives (green or black): 8

Calorie-reduced sources (approximately 25 calories a portion)

Light tub margarine: 1 tsp.

Light cream cheese: 1 tsp.

Fat-free salad dressing: 1 TB.

Snack Time

Snacking seems to be increasing, especially for runners who need to keep themselves constantly fueled. Use caution when snacking, especially if you're trying to lose weight; every calorie needs to be accounted for.

Snacks are just fractions of meal size, and it has to be "smart food" or "fuel" for your competitive and physiological fire. You can snack too much or not smart enough if you take in too many useless calories.

Drink, Drink—and Then Drink Some More

Runners need to drink lots of water (at least eight large glasses a day) and eat lots of fruits and vegetables. Athletes who drink plenty of water tend to consume fewer total calories than those who don't drink as much.

If you fill up on water and high-water-content drinks and foods (such as cucumbers, tomatoes, lettuce, peaches, and so on), you'll be less likely to eat foods that are bad for you. Water is the preferred beverage when trying to lose or maintain ideal body weight.

Supplementation

It is estimated that nearly 40 percent of Americans use supplements today. That's big business! There are also close to 30,000 supplements to choose from, and many manufacturers and advertisers claim miraculous new discoveries will improve your health. Many times, the old adage of "if it sounds to good to be true, it probably is" is correct, but there are supplements that are proven and are certainly worth taking.

> **Watch Your Step**
>
> The following is a great mixture of supplements that work together in warding off anemia and fatigue. I have used this combination for the athletes I train with great success: Mix 1 milligram folic acid with 8 ounces of orange juice and a 500-milligram tablet of vitamin C (finely crushed); add 1 teaspoon ferrous sulfate elixir (liquid iron). Drink 30 minutes before breakfast. Drinking before your meal is important, because you want the most effective absorption rate possible.

The Food and Drug Administration (FDA) does not regulate supplements; they do not fall into the food category, and they are not classified as drugs. This lack of governance has allowed advertisers to make claims about their products that are untrue or go unproven at best, and it is difficult if not impossible to know the purity of the products and if the dosage recommended is correct.

Eat More (Often), Lose More (Weight)

Many runners who are trying to lose or maintain their body weight need to eat smaller meals five times a day. This idea has led the supplement industry to create products such as energy bars and meal-replacement drinks. Energy bars are a good way to get in a meal between breakfast, lunch, and dinner. Be sure to drink plenty of water with your energy bar to help with digestion. Energy bars can be good alternatives for athletes "on the go" who would otherwise not eat or would eat something not nearly as nutritious.

Athletes who have a hard time eating breakfast may try a meal-replacement mix or an energy bar instead of not eating. Not eating breakfast will slow your basal metabolism rate, and more than likely you will end up eating some nonessential calories later on. Meal-replacement mixes are usually high in protein and low in fat and can be mixed with water or juice. These mixes can provide a great source of fuel and are a great way to get a quick meal in.

One of the largest parts of the supplement business is a fluid-replacement drink. It is very important to remember that there is no replacement for proper hydration with water. Don't allow your body to become thirsty; this is the signal that your body is already dehydrated.

Intake: Timing Is Everything

If you want to drink a fluid other than water before or during your run, be sure that the carbohydrate solution is 6 percent or less. This will allow the fluid to be absorbed quickly into your bloodstream and will help your body not to lose performance. Also be sure that the source of carbohydrates is coming from complex carbohydrates (maltodextrin), not simple sugars (fructose, sucrose, dextrose, glucose).

Runner Facts

The best way to take vitamin B_{12} is by a sublingual (under your tongue) pill. Studies show that this method allows the best absorption rate possible.

After your run, you have a two-hour window when the body will replenish glycogen (stored carbohydrates) a little more effectively. These drinks also offer many electrolytes and high-carbohydrate ingredients to help the body recover from exercise. Like always, make sure that these carbohydrates are complex and not simple ones.

Gel packs seem to be the rage with long-endurance runners today. They provide the same types of energy replacement as fluid-replacement drinks without all the water content. This can be a good source of energy for a long workout or a good way to meet that two-hour window when trying to replenish quickly. Also, if you're a runner who prefers water to fluid-replacement drinks, this may be the product for you.

Most runners who adhere to a well-balanced diet will not need many supplements. Many runners who take supplements are wasting their money on "overkill," taking much larger doses than necessary—or they are taking supplements with erroneous claims.

When Should You Take Supplements?

Who benefits from nutritional supplements? Here are a few reasons why a person would take supplements:

◆ **Runners training in harsh environments.** Runners training at altitude will need to take additional iron, as they will have a larger red blood cell count than the normal person or runner training at sea level. Also, runners training in extreme heat or extreme cold will need to take supplements to keep their immune systems strong.

◆ **Female athletes.** To prevent anemia, runners need iron as they lose iron through menstruation. Iron aids the blood and oxygen transportation system; being low in iron will severely limit your ability to run well.

◆ **Female athletes not menstruating.** Female runners who are not menstruating have a greater need for calcium. There is a much higher incidence of stress fractures with women who are not menstruating versus those who are.

◆ **Runners who are dieting.** If you are restricting your total caloric intake to less than 1,400 calories, you may be missing some essential vitamins and nutrients that are important for your overall health.

◆ **Runners who are vegetarians.** Cutting meat out of your diet severely limits your likelihood of getting enough iron, zinc, vitamins D and B_{12}, and riboflavin.

◆ **Pregnant runners.** Pay special attention to your physician's advice on prenatal supplementation. Usually this advice will include supplementing iron and folic acid, as well as taking a prenatal multivitamin.

◆ **Runners who are lactose intolerant.** Athletes who cannot eat dairy products will likely fall short of meeting their calcium and riboflavin needs.

◆ **Runners who have food allergies.** When you cut out a food group or a series of foods, you will have a harder time getting all the essential vitamins and nutrients you need.

◆ **Runners who want to boost performance (legally!).** Many runners should take calcium, as it increases bone density and can prevent cramps and aid in muscle recovery. Any one of these reasons would be adequate, but collectively it is an essential mineral to think about taking.

What Supplements Should You Take?

Here is a list of supplements commonly used by runners. This list is not all-inclusive, but rather a guide of commonly used supplements:

calcium   Strengthens bones and aids in muscle contractions during exercise.

carbohydrate   Provides the best energy sources for your body.

chromium   Helps your cells process carbohydrates for energy.

fish oil   Assists in lowering blood cholesterol and has anti-inflammatory benefits.

folic acid Helps keep red blood cells healthy and serves as an aid in preventing anemia.

glucosamine and chondroitin sulfate Used as an anti-inflammatory to ease inflammation and joint pain.

iron Aids the blood in oxygen transportation to your muscles.

magnesium Assists the body in aerobic capacity and plays a critical role in endurance performance.

protein Helps alleviate fatigue and aids the injury recovery process.

sodium bicarbonate (baking soda) Aids the body in buffering lactic acid.

vitamin B$_{12}$ Plays an important role in the production of red blood cells and helps break carbohydrates down into glucose.

vitamin C Very important in maintaining a strong immune system.

vitamin E Antioxidant that assists in preventing muscle soreness.

zinc Immune booster; aids athletes in their ability to fight off illness and infections.

Finding Your Healthy Body Weight

How does body weight fit into your goal of running injury-free? Actually, it ties in perfectly. Don't let your weight consume you, but don't consume so much of the wrong stuff that your weight becomes all-consuming either.

As a coach, I am always trying to figure out a way to keep my athletes healthy, injury-free, and—of course—racing fast. One topic that always comes up is weight—what is their ideal training weight, and what is their ideal racing weight.

Many of you probably started running in the first place to lose weight. It's not surprising; in today's society, our body size and weight has become increasingly more important because of marketing images. But more

Runner Facts

As a result of our image-conscious society, half of all American women and nearly 25 percent of men are trying to lose weight.

important than that TV-image body is the need to take care of yourself and lead a healthy lifestyle, so that the years you have left are truly quality ones.

Considering how many people are dieting, it's clear this is big money, so it's no wonder that there are so many fad diets and plans.

What's Right for Me?

First thing's first: is there an "ideal" body weight? Many self-appointed "gurus" out there will tell you that if you are a certain height, you should be a certain weight. I contend that since everyone has different genetics, goals, and objectives, your "ideal" body weight will be a very individual issue.

We all are very different; we all have our own unique muscle and bone structure. If you love the way you look, that's good, because genetics are non-negotiable. And if you don't like it, no matter how much you might want to change, you will need to consider your genes in your overall plan. If you try to starve yourself and take shortcuts in addressing your body weight, you will be injured in no time. Having said that, here are some principles that I hope will help you achieve *your* perfect weight.

Your Ideal Weight

There are three distinct body types—see if you can find yours in these descriptions. If you're tall and thin and find it hard to gain weight or muscle, you're an *ectomorph*. Depending on your leg speed, you may be able to race well at anything from the 5k to the marathon and stay injury-free. As you have probably guessed, many world-class runners fit this type. If you're muscular with stocky arms and legs, you are a *mesomorph*. Again, depending on your leg speed, mesomorphs tend to make great sprinters and sometimes run middle distances well. Lastly, if you have a little more body fat and your body is more round, you're an *endomorph*. The endomorph is usually a weight or throws type of athlete. If you find yourself in the "larger" category, don't despair. Many current races have a "Clydesdale division"—which might be a perfect fit for someone who has a few pounds to lose or is just starting out.

Let's look at how your training needs to be adjusted based on your body type. If you're an ectomorph, you're a good candidate for a higher mileage program with no repercussions. But this type of distance training isn't for the mesomorph or endomorph—it's too much pounding on your legs and joints. These types need to lower their mileage and run on soft surfaces, with the proper support and cushioned running shoe. Once you adjust your training program to your body type, you're much less likely to have an injury related to size and weight issues.

> **Runner Facts**
>
> Is anyone really just one body type? Probably not. Most of us are a combination of two or three. Let's just hope you get the parts that complement each other! Knowing your type will help you pick a training program that keeps you healthy and competitive.

Maintaining and Losing Weight the Right Way

To estimate your daily caloric needs for maintaining your current body weight, take your current weight and multiply it by 13. This is the number of calories per day that will maintain your present weight. That will cover your basal metabolism and enough extra calories for easy activities. So if you weigh 160 pounds, you will need about 2,080 calories per day to maintain your present weight at your current activity level.

> **Watch Your Step**
>
> To lose 1 pound each week, you must then create a deficit of 500 calories a day for 7 days, as 3,500 calories equals 1 pound of weight.

Then you must decide how you much weight you want to lose. Most nutritionists suggest losing no more than 1 to 2 pounds a week for the normal person. To lose 1 pound, you need to have a deficit of 500 calories per day. The amount of calories you cut from your nutritional program depends a lot on how many calories you're consuming now.

Continued weight loss will be a lot easier to manage as you add in your training. Running 1 mile will equal approximately 100 calories of caloric expenditure. So if a 160-pound runner runs 5 miles (500-calorie expenditure) and eats 2,080 calories every day, he would lose 1 pound per week. Or you can eat 250 fewer calories (1,830 a day) and run 2½ miles per day to come up with the deficit of 500 per day. Remember, most experts recommend a loss of no more than 2 pounds per week, as this will cause breakdown of muscle tissue.

In Their Shoes

In the summer of 2007, I met a young man from Texas; he came into my office with one of my former athletes and introduced himself. He looked tall and lean, with a very typical runner's body type. Yet when he went into his personal story, I realized the journey he took to my office was anything but typical.

After high school athletics, in which he had excelled, he attended a Division I university where he was part of the running program. He didn't do well—in fact, you could say it chewed him up and spit him out. With his confidence gone, he quit school and walked away from training. He didn't see a use for it and couldn't fit training and working out into his lifestyle.

Before long, he began to smoke. Next came fast food and too many desserts. He found himself gaining weight and before he knew it, he had ballooned from a fit 150 pounds to over 220. At first he was in denial about how the extra weight was affecting him. Heck, he just looked more like a football player than a runner. But quickly the health consequences of gaining so much weight in such a short time period set in.

About a year after he gained so much weight, he found himself short of breath on a trip. And not just any trip; it was a short jaunt from the couch to the refrigerator. He knew that was it; he had to regain control of his weight and his life. He began by walking short distances at fairly slow paces. Once he could do this without shortness of breath, he started to jog. He could only maintain the running for 200 yards and then he would return to walking. Over time, he increased the running portion of his workout, and after a few months, he could run a mile without walking. A year later, he had done it: he weighed 155 and felt like an athlete again.

He continued his fitness quest and regained some confidence and courage. He came to my office that summer with a goal: would I allow him to walk on to my cross-country team and see if he could make it? A brave goal for a 25-year-old with this type of life experience.

I welcomed him, and this fall he will attempt to make the cross-country team and—more important—will get back into school and pursue a degree. I don't know how it will all turn out, but regardless of how his competitive experience goes, he's already a winner in my eyes.

Losing weight is extremely difficult compared to putting it on (except for those darn ectomorphs), but you can do it by following a healthy routine. Don't let those fad diets and supplements fool you. If you want to lose weight, there are no shortcuts. This plan will keep you running and injury-free whether you're maintaining weight or losing those few extra pounds.

Dr. Ernst Van Aaken, a noted physiologist and philosopher, once said, "Eat as if you were a poor man, do endurance training daily, and don't let your mind go to seed." This is still great advice, especially in the today's world of fast food, overeating, and indulgence in all things sweet. It takes a little discipline, but the results will keep you feeling great and running strong.

Effects of Weight Gain

Increasing your weight will lower your VO2 Max. This will have a dramatic effect on your training and racing performances, as well as adding to the pounding that your body takes with every step. It takes over 1,000 strides to run a mile, so extra pounds you carry will lead to fatigue and greater risk of injury. Take a 1,500-meter run for example: gaining 1 kilogram (2.2 lb.) of weight can slow your performance down as much as 4 to 7 seconds for an elite runner and as much as 10 to 12 seconds for a beginner. Over a longer race, this can translate to much larger numbers—a minute or more for 5ks and 10ks.

Performing Successfully at All Weights

The media is constantly sending mixed messages to the American public. On one hand, the message is that fat is bad and you need to avoid it; on the other hand, you need to be comfortable with your body size and makeup. Certainly we know obesity is not healthy, but we all need some fat to run well for endurance races.

The perception is that you must be anorexic to run fast, but if you're trying to lose weight by reducing too many calories per day and still continuing to run normally, you can and will most likely begin to develop sickness and injury problems. These problems usually begin as colds and normal fatigue and can advance to more serious problems like amenorrhea (women not having menstrual periods), muscle problems, and osteoporosis. You're better off eating a well-balanced diet with proper nutrients (vitamins and minerals), and not having to deal with chronic fatigue, colds, flu, and stress fractures.

Running as a Weight-Loss Tool

Losing weight is hard work, and for some people it seems like no matter which diet they try, the weight just hangs on. Sometimes to truly lose weight we need to get back to the basics—eat a better diet and increase our level of exercise.

No matter which way you go, the basics are the same. You need to burn more calories than you consume to have a net reduction in your weight. If you are looking to running as a tool in your weight-loss program, you're off to a good start. Writing down what you eat and how much exercise you get each day is a great way to get a good perspective on your net gain/loss. Did you burn more calories than you took in?

Eating breakfast helps jump-start your body and gets your metabolism going strong. Increasing the amount of fruits and vegetables you take in will also help. You need protein and carbohydrates to give you energy, especially as you train, so keep them at a higher proportion of your total food intake.

Stay active—running burns calories, and lots of them. Once you establish a training program, stick with it. If you find yourself stuck in a weight-loss stage, adjust your workout. Add a little more mileage or do your current mileage with a greater intensity. Either way, you will kick up your body's metabolism, which in turn will lead to greater weight loss.

Weigh yourself once a week; more than that and your body doesn't have time to produce results. Once you begin to see the pounds dropping, that weekly weigh-in will keep you motivated in your training. Always weigh yourself without clothes and fully hydrated.

Road Blocks

Even highly motivated runners experience problems maintaining performance when dieting. If you're struggling to lose weight and you're not performing well, re-evaluate your plan. Maybe it's not realistic, or maybe you need to eat more and worry less about your genetic makeup.

No matter what you think your ideal weight should be, if you're restricting your caloric intake and having health issues and injuries, you need to consider an alternate plan. These are warning signs, so you need to listen to your body.

You may not have the talent to break a world record, but you certainly can achieve high goals and improvement if you're willing to take the time and do the work. If you have gained weight and are struggling to run times you ran a year ago, establish a seasonal best time and set your sights on getting better. Changing your mindset will allow you to break up the big picture and focus on the smaller tasks of getting to where you need to be.

The Least You Need to Know

◆ When you eat is often as important as what you eat.

◆ You gained weight eating too much, and you'll lose it eating less—and training.

◆ You've got to know what you are eating—if it's a carb, fat, or protein.

◆ Genetics play a big role—play the hand you were dealt.

Chapter 6

Warming Up and Cooling Down

In This Chapter

- ◆ Why the warm-up is so often overlooked
- ◆ Why warming up is so important and helps prevent injuries
- ◆ When and where the warm-up and cooldown fit into your routine
- ◆ How to measure a successful warm-up and cooldown by heart rate

One of the most overlooked aspects of staying healthy as a runner—I would argue the *most* often ignored—is the proper warm-up and cooldown.

The heart and other muscles do a lot of work. Trying to jump right in without a proper warm-up can set you up for injury, and failing to cool down takes your heart rate from all-out to sedentary.

Making Time for Warming and Cooling

When I first arrived at Adams State College, I began my job with a very small group of about eight young women who didn't have much of a clue about what college running was all about. You see, the men had traditionally dominated the program and the women's team was not at the same level. We had a few very talented athletes, but no true team to speak of.

I began my first day with a new set of warm-ups and stretches that I had used during my running career. About 20 minutes later, we had completed the warm-up. When I suggested that we were now ready for our workout, the expressions on their faces said it all—they thought the workout had ended. Several commented that they had never run or stretched that much before and were now too tired to train. Needless to say, I had to regroup, provide some education, and slowly move this team toward a true training program. We got there eventually, once they got into shape and learned how to work out properly; we were on our way to a first-place finish at the national championship.

I share that story with you because I think it is important to train both your body and your mind on the different elements of a well-rounded running program. Warming up, workouts and/or races, and cooling down should go hand in hand. One without the others is a recipe for a wide variety of injuries.

If you have always been one of those runners who call the first 10 minutes of your run your "warm-up" and the last 10 minutes your "cooldown," then at least be sure you are doing it correctly and not causing yourself any potential injury. Learn the basics of warming up and cooling down the right way. Furthermore, be consistent in the way you implement these into your program—it only takes once to be sorry you didn't.

Joints: Chiefs of Movement Staff

Why is warming up so important? So you're motivated and ready get out the door and start running; you're excited to get fit so you can feel better and have more energy. Before you jump into your full training regimen, you need to learn a few basic principles of how and why to warm up and cool down properly.

Have you ever started out a run and wondered why your joints feel like they won't move? Or maybe you feel like you can't lift your legs or arms until well into the workout? Both of these are symptoms of the lack of a proper warm-up period. Running with cold muscles that do not absorb the impact is uncomfortable as well as a potential injury, as the colder muscle is more susceptible to pulls and strains. Properly warmed-up muscles will allow you greater range of motion in your joints, enabling you to run faster and with better form.

Most runners can recognize the benefits of getting their aching muscles to loosen up and flow before raising the intensity of their run. Build up to a hard workout with a planned warm-up—without overdoing it.

Even the Best Plan Might Need Adapting

I took my team to the prestigious Penn Relays in 2007. It is quite a track meet—actually, I would call it *the* track meet myself. A huge number of athletes participate, while thousands of spectators enjoy track and field racing at its finest. As a very small school at high altitude, we don't get to attend meets of this caliber very often, so every runner knows that when we have the opportunity to race at sea level, we must make the most of it.

At a meet like this, the management does its best to run each event on time; needless to say, timing is everything. Athletes warm up on the streets of Philadelphia or find a nearby park. Once the runners are called, they proceed to a paddock area jam-packed with athletes preparing to run. After you enter this area, your warm-up usually comes to a screeching halt. Coaches and athletes alike are warned that the meet is on a tight schedule and you must be ready at the exact time or risk missing your event.

On the first day, our first relay team was warmed up and ready to go at exactly the minute the schedule called for, but—lo and behold—Mother Nature had a different plan and dumped rain by the buckets. A long rain delay set the schedule back by almost an hour. As the new race time approached, the warm-ups began again, and we finally ran the race.

My athletes didn't perform nearly as well as any of us thought they would. They looked a little flat, not up to their normal racing levels. After considering all the factors that impacted the race that day,

I believe the delay and the "over warm-up" had a negative effect. All teams had the same set of circumstances; I just think I made an error in allowing my team to warm up too early. As the old saying goes, live and learn.

As you prepare for a hard interval workout or maybe a race that you are peaking toward, be sure you factor in timing as part of your workout routine. Remember, there is a delicate balance between not warming up enough and warming up too much.

What the Warm-Up Is ... and Isn't

The "warm-up" is a preventative measure to reduce the risk of injury. And while this is the primary reason you should do your warm-up, there are other great benefits as well. These benefits include giving you a high-quality hard session, since your heart is prepared for the upcoming workout, and better range of motion, as your muscles are looser and more pliable. Starting to run slowly and allowing your muscles to increase the amount of blood in your tissues, slowly increasing the oxygen going to your working muscles, will make your muscles more pliable and resistant to injury.

> **Runner Facts**
>
> A proper warm-up will help you mentally prepare for the hard workout ahead. Doing a more specific warm-up can prepare your neuromuscular system for a good fast race or interval session.

How do I go about warming up correctly? To be sure your warm-up is sufficient, start running easy and slowly progress until your heart rate reaches 120 to 140 beats per minute. Your breathing should also increase, allowing you to oxygenate all your working muscles and slightly increase the temperature of your active muscles. It is a good sign that you have warmed up properly if you have broken into a mild sweat.

I ensure that my athletes warm up for all of their runs, even on easy days. I truly believe that over the years this has diminished the number and severity of injuries we incur. So even if you're warming up to go for that easy run, allow 10 to 15 minutes for your pre-run warm-up.

Better Warm-Up Equals Better Results

I require that my athletes do a much longer warm-up if they are getting ready for a hard interval session or a race. Experiment in your practices to see what works best for you. I believe young runners tend to underdo the warm-up, feeling that it is unnecessary, or they're rushed, or they feel that a longer, more appropriate warm-up may tire them out. I teach them that warming up correctly will only boost their performance and keep them healthy.

What are the differences between warming up for an easy day versus a hard workout or race? The easy-day warm-up: begin with five minutes of easy jogging, starting very slow and progressing until you've broken a sweat. Then I have a series of stretches that I suggest you complete on easy days. (We'll get very detailed about stretching in the next chapter.) If you don't have time for both this warm-up and your run, be sure to start your run very slowly and only progress to faster running when you're sure your joints and muscles are fully warmed up.

On hard days or race days: start with easier jogging—10 to 15 minutes or so—then take another 10 to 15 minutes to stretch. After you stretch, do three to five progressively faster strides to stimulate your central nervous system and wake up dormant fast-twitch muscle fibers. This particular warm-up will enable you to have that great workout or race.

Steps to a Proper Warm-Up

Think of warming up and cooling down in the following 10 steps. Do a few easy stretches. Try moving your arms around, bending over and flexing the large muscles in your body. Move to holding each major stretch for about 20 to 30 seconds each. Begin to jog slowly. Easy on the running, though: the point is to loosen up.

Continue the jog for about five to eight minutes. Walk briskly if you feel too stiff to jog at the beginning. Stop. Stretch fully. The stretching will feel easier and you will notice that your muscles are warm. Stretch each muscle group, starting at the top of your body and moving down. Loosen your shoulders, neck, arms, quads, hamstrings, and calves. Stretch your Achilles.

Start your run, slow and easy, building into the hard workout phase. At the completion of your hard phase, begin the slow-down process again. Cool down. Jog and then walk for the last five to eight minutes to allow a good return for the blood flow. Perform a few ending stretches.

The Cooldown

Cooling down gradually after your run is critical to your recovery and sets you up to have a great run the next day. A gradual cooldown will return your heart rate and breathing patterns to normal, helping you avoid fainting or dizziness. Stopping instantly after a hard session causes blood to pool in your active muscles and doesn't allow the blood in your working muscles to be redispersed gradually back to your organs (heart and brain).

In Their Shoes

Why is it important to cool down? When I was competing in road races earlier in my career, I would see runners finishing a race, pulling on some sweats, changing shoes (maybe), and heading off to their cars. They might grab some water (it was water in paper cups back then, before we saw the need to buy it in the bottle), drink some, and then pour the rest over their head.

At one race, I remember that after most of the participants had finished, I was cooling down and rounded a corner just in time to see a man collapse to the ground. I ran over to help as he was trying to pull himself back up. He said he felt dizzy and faint, that things starting spinning and before he knew what happened, he was on the ground.

While everything turned out okay in this case, it was a great lesson to me about the need to cool down properly. If you abruptly stop running after a hard effort, you, too, could risk this fate.

Cooling down properly will allow you to remove the metabolic waste products that have accumulated in your muscles during your run, such as lactic acid. Ridding your blood of these waste by-products prepares your muscles for the next exercise session, either the next day or several days later. I also believe that a proper cooldown will reduce postworkout muscle soreness.

The Mechanics of a Proper Cooldown

You will need to gradually slow down your running pace over 5 to 15 minutes. A harder run or workout requires a longer cooldown because these produce larger quantities of metabolic waste in your blood. If you had a relative easy run, you only need to gradually slow down your run over the last 5 to 10 minutes.

It's best to stretch following your workout, as this allows you to get rid of any kinks or tightness that developed during your run. If at all possible, stretch all your body parts (arms, legs, midsection, back, and so on). Stretching after you run should only take an additional 10 minutes. If you're pressed for time, at least stretch your legs and back, as they take the most beating during your run. The legs are also the most prone to injury and stretching will help prevent problems, restoring your muscles to their resting length and improve flexibility. It will also help increase the range of motion in your joints.

A proper cooldown will help lower the possibility of cramping, muscle soreness, and muscle stiffness.

Ice: The Really Cool Option

The principles of icing are as basic as the body's healing processes. In very simple terms, it is about the muscles, tendons, bones, nerves, and tissues recovering from a hard workout or race.

As we talked about in Chapter 4 on energy, the body produces lactic acid, a waste product of exercise. When you build too much of this lactic acid, your muscles develop a feeling of fatigue, and with runners in particular, you can have that heavy-legged feeling.

When you submerge your legs in an ice bath after a hard workout or race, the cold water causes your blood vessels to tighten up and push the blood out of your legs. After 5 to 10 minutes, your legs will begin to feel very cold and numb.

Ice baths invigorate the legs and stimulate blood flow for healing. The ice nips any bleeding that you have in muscle and other tissues before it progresses into an injury. Once you exit the ice bath, your legs will begin to fill back up with fresh blood, stimulating your muscles with oxygen and helping the cells function better. At the same time, the old blood will carry away the lactic acid and cleanse the legs.

In Their Shoes

About 10 years ago, I really began to see the benefits of ice as a healing agent. We were visited in Alamosa by a team of international athletes who brought their own entourage to assist them in preparing for the New York City Marathon.

One of the trainers who came along on the trip had a background in horseracing and had several interesting techniques. As I learned the physiology behind his methods, I decided to incorporate them into my own training program.

After some horses finish a workout or a race, the trainers use cold compresses to stimulate the animals' legs. This allows the blood to flow back into the main part of the cavity and uses the cold as healing agent. I figured that if it was good enough for million-dollar racehorses, it was good enough for Adams State College runners.

Be careful when you get out of an ice bath. You legs will be wobbly, so watch your step. The ideal temperature of an ice bath is around 45 to 50°F—cool enough to be effective, but not so cold that it freezes the skin. The best type of ice bath is a whirlpool designed for soaking the body or legs. But in the absence of this, you can use a cold-water bathtub or place cold towels on your legs while leaning them against the wall or propping them up higher than you heart.

Contrast Showers

A popular way to get some benefits from cold water is to use the contrasting shower methods. After you complete a workout or even perhaps as your regular morning shower, try alternating between hot and cold water.

Begin showering and then alternate between 1 minute of warm water and 1 minute of cold water, for 8 to 10 minutes. The contrast in temperature promotes blood flow and stimulates the nervous system, both of which positively influence recovery and arousal levels and help the healing and blood transfer process.

No matter what your method, make warming up and cooling down part of your program and your daily routine. It's right up there with stretching—as important to your muscles and your heart as stretching is to your muscles and your joints. It only takes a little time to properly warm up and cool down, yet the time it saves you is huge.

In the next chapter, you can find a whole menu of great stretches.

The Least You Need to Know

- The warm-up is more than just the first part of your run.

- Failing to warm up and cool down properly is one of the big mistakes runners make—sometimes even elite runners, but especially young and novice runners.

- The cooldown is not the last five minutes of your run; it's an actual program to bring down the heart rate and cool your body machine.

- Ice is still a relatively untapped gold mine in the restorative process.

Chapter 7

Stretching ... the Truth

In This Chapter

- ◆ How proper stretching relates to biomechanics
- ◆ The difference between static and dynamic stretching
- ◆ When the proper time to stretch is—and isn't
- ◆ Why tight muscles are a precursor of potential injuries
- ◆ What the proper stretches are, and how to do them

When you get out of a car after a long ride, or stand up after sitting at a desk several hours, you can feel the tightness going through your body. This stiff, sluggish feeling reminds you how inflexible you can become after even just a few hours without having range of motion.

Gaining knowledge about stretching and flexibility will help you stay injury-free and improve your overall fitness. I am a strong believer in stretching and flexibility training. I have seen over and over how athletes who have better range of motion are able to use this to their advantage in competition and training, allowing themselves to run faster and remain healthy.

When you run and work out, you build muscle tissue, and as that muscle builds, it can become shorter (tighter). You therefore need to work at lengthening the muscle, as well as your tendons and Achilles, to have the best chance to remain injury-free. Stretching helps your body begin to loosen up and prepare itself for the workout, which allows you to get more out of your biomechanics during the training session. Improving your flexibility and coordination increases your overall health and fitness.

Let's first learn about the different types of stretching.

Static Stretching

This method of stretching involves extending a muscle or group of muscles until you feel that good stretch, and then holding that position for a time interval. Most athletes can do static stretching, and it's considered one of the safest methods of stretching.

When performed correctly, static stretching requires a small expenditure of energy and allows adequate rest to reset the muscle before the next stretch. It assists in lengthening the muscle and can aid you in relaxing your muscles as well.

Most static exercises guide you to do two to five repetitions and hold the stretches for 10 to 30 seconds each.

Dynamic Stretching

Dynamic stretching is most often associated with warming up. It involves gentle, progressive movements that build gradual intensity over time. One of the primary purposes of dynamic stretching is improving joint mobility.

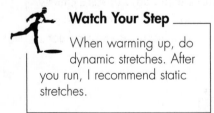

Watch Your Step

When warming up, do dynamic stretches. After you run, I recommend static stretches.

You begin these types of stretches with limited range of movements and build up to full joint movement. It does not involve any type of bouncing movements within the stretches. Dynamic stretching should be performed in repetitions, generally sets of 8 to 10.

Ballistic Stretching

This type of stretching involves pushing the body beyond its normal range of motion. It is controversial and limited in its benefits to runners. The types of movements involved are often bouncing, bobbing, jumping, lunging, and rebounding.

The drawbacks of this type of stretching are that it does not give your body adequate time to adapt to the movement and can increase your risk of injury. For specific types of workouts (martial arts, for example) it can be beneficial, but I suggest staying away from this type of stretching in your running program.

Active Stretching

When you do active stretching, you perform movements by assuming a stretching position and maintaining it without any assistance or equipment. An example would be lifting your leg up and holding it in that position with nothing except the strength of your leg muscle.

This type of stretching improves flexibility and strengthens your body. These types of stretches are common in various forms of yoga and generally require you to hold the stretch 10 to 15 seconds, with several repetitions.

Passive Stretching

This is the opposite of active stretching. An external force is applied, either by a partner or piece of equipment. This type of stretching can be very effective when the muscle in question is weak or you need to stretch beyond your normal range.

When working with a partner, it is important to communicate clearly to prevent the muscle from being pushed too far and thus injured. These types of stretches are often used in team settings or in rehabilitation situations.

When and How to Stretch

You've probably been wondering when and how to fit stretching and flexibility into your complete training program. I believe that you should tie as much of it as possible to your regular running workout, but there are benefits if you do stretching and flexibility training at other times.

Incorporate some stretches into your warm-up before you run. They will help loosen your muscles and get your engine ready for the workout. But after your workout is the best time to incorporate more comprehensive stretches and flexibility exercises. Right after you work out, your body is warm and pliable. You have an increased range of motion, so this is a great opportunity to get the most out of your flexibility work and keep your muscles from fighting back.

Keeping variety in your stretching and flexibility routine will help keep you engaged and enjoying it. If you fall into that easy routine of doing the same stretches and flexibility program each time, you eventually become less intense and effective, and the benefits of your efforts decrease.

One strategy for adding variety is to occasionally find a partner and do different stretches and flexibility exercises together. The company will add some spice and help you push yourself differently.

In Their Shoes

Ryan came into our program with great high school marks and embraced the Adams State training fully. Well, almost. He did an excellent job of training on the track and road, and he began a lifting program to try and improve his strength and speed. He improved his cardiovascular fitness and he could certainly lift more—but his performances weren't getting any better. As a matter of fact, at several meets he was just dismal.

I sat Ryan down and tried to analyze what was going on. We even did some testing and found that his stride length had decreased. What could be causing this? Then it clicked—Ryan had added a great deal of weight training into his program, but hadn't seen the benefits of flexibility training or stretching. As a result of this imbalanced workout, his muscles had bound up—contracted—and were actually inhibiting his range of motion and impacting his performance.

Right away we began a regiment of stretching and flexibility work. He incorporated this into his training program with the same vigor he brought to the other aspects of his training, and the results soon came. Ryan got back to his old performance standards and eventually went on to set personal bests and win races.

Only a comprehensive, balanced approach will keep you injury-free and give you the results you seek!

The rest of this chapter lists a menu of stretches you can pick from and use to build your own stretching and flexibility program. You should use some of them almost daily; others you can use when you have tightness in a particular area.

Upper Body

From shoulder and arm stretches to arm circles, the following are great stretches for your upper body.

Shoulder and Arm Stretch

1. Stand with your feet as wide as your hips.

2. Relax and hang your arms down beside your body.

3. Raise one arm as if you are trying to reach the ceiling. The other arm remains hanging down. Hold this position for 15 seconds.

4. Drop your arm back down. Repeat.

5. Change to your alternate arm. Repeat the exercise. Do three to five repetitions.

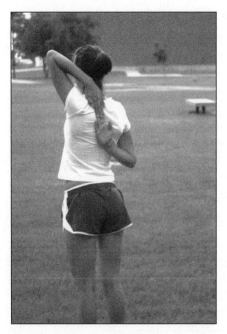

This stretch is good for the shoulder and upper back.

Upper Back Stretch

1. Stand up straight, knees slightly bent, feet placed even with your hips, and toes pointed forward.

2. Extend both your arms, forming a 90-degree angle between your body and arms.

3. Bring your hands forward until they point directly out in front of you.

4. Clasp you hands together, palms facing forward, and hold. You will feel the stretch in your upper back. Hold the stretch for six to eight seconds.

A variation of this stretch is repeating the process while sitting in a straight chair.

Shoulder/Upper Back Stretch

1. Sit in a chair or stand with a straight back. Keep both feet on the floor and your weight evenly balanced.

2. Take your left hand and gently place it on your right shoulder blade, palm facing down.

3. With your other arm, reach to your back and try to connect your fingers. Do this without arching your back or pushing out your chest. (Don't worry if your fingers don't touch. As your flexibility improves, so will your reach.) Hold for 10 seconds.

4. Repeat five times.

5. Switch arms and repeat.

Neck Stretch

1. Sit in a chair. Place the palm of your hand on the crown of your head.

2. Lower your chin toward your chest without leaning forward and gently press your head back against your hand while your hand

provides resistance against your head. Keep your head straight and try looking at your foot as a focal point. Hold for 15 seconds and release.

3. Repeat four times.

4. Switch to the other side and opposite hand; repeat.

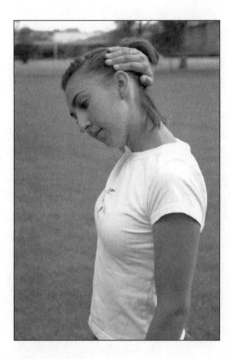

Stretching the neck is easy but important.

Arm Stretch Against Wall

1. Stand beside a wall, approximately 1 foot away from the wall. Reach up with your arm, placing your hand on the wall, palm side toward the wall.

2. Lean into the wall. Hold for 15 seconds.

3. Repeat five times.

4. Switch sides and repeat.

Arm Circles

1. Stand with your arms at a 90-degree angle from your body, palms facing forward. Your body will form a T.

2. Begin by making small circles with your hands, then increase the size of the circles until you are using your complete arms range of motion. Complete 10 circles.

3. Repeat with your palms facing back.

4. Repeat the stretch by reversing (moving backward) the direction of your arm circles.

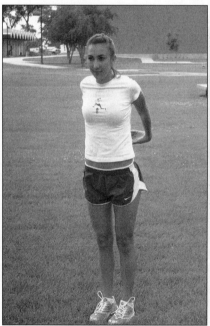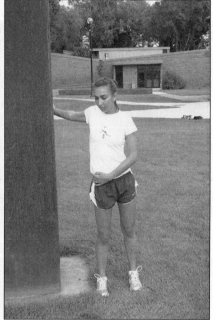

Either of these chest stretches gets the job done.

Chest Stretch

1. Stand up straight, slightly bent at the knees. Place your feet even with your hips, toes pointing forward.

2. Place your arms behind your back. Keeping your shoulders level, clasp your hands together and hold.

3. Breathe in through your nose, then exhale out of your mouth while holding this stretch for six to eight seconds.

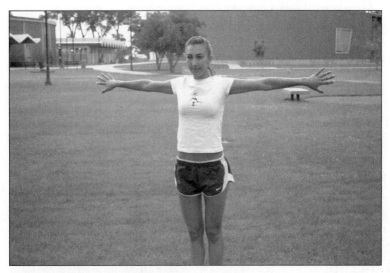

A quick and easy bicep stretch.

Bicep Stretch

1. Lift your arms to the side, bringing them to shoulder height, forming a 90-degree with the side of your body. Your body will form a T.

2. Rotate your wrists to the point where your palms face behind you.

3. Push back with your arms until you feel the stretch in your upper arms. Hold stretch for six to eight seconds.

Triceps Stretch

1. Stand up straight, knees slightly bent, feet placed even with your hips, and toes pointed forward.

2. Bend your right arm at the elbow, lifting your arm next to your head. Have your right fingers touch your shoulder blade area.

3. Place your left arm across the top of your head, touching your right elbow.

4. Push back on your elbow until you feel your triceps stretch. Hold for 10 seconds.

5. Repeat with the other arm.

Triceps are the bigger of the two arm muscles.

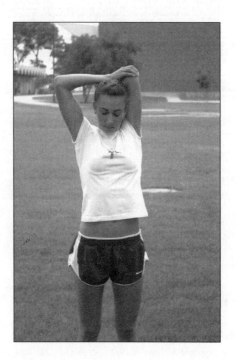

Cross Shoulder Stretch

1. Stand up straight, knees slightly bent, feet placed even with your hips, and toes pointed forward.

2. Bend your right arm at the elbow and extend it across your chest.

3. Place your left hand on the back side of your right elbow and pull your arm across your body until you feel your right upper arm and shoulder stretch. Hold for six to eight seconds.

4. Repeat the stretch, switching arms.

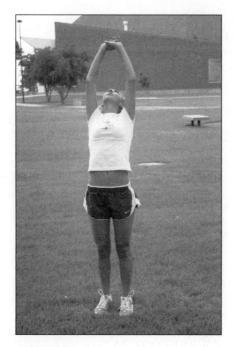

This full-body stretch works wonders.

Full-Body Stretch

1. Stand upright with your feet even with your shoulders and hips.

2. Slowly lift both arms out to your side and then up over your head.

3. Clasp your hands and reach for the stars. Feel the muscles in your entire body lengthen and stretch out. Hold for 10 to 15 seconds.

4. Repeat five times.

Middle Body

From groin stretches to hip flexor stretches, the following are great stretches for your middle body.

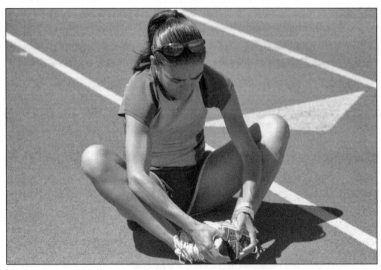

The groin muscle must be stretched every workout.

Groin Stretch

1. Begin the groin stretch by sitting on the floor with the soles of your feet together, your back straight, your head up, and your elbows on the insides of your knees.

2. Place your arms across your legs and grab your feet, then slowly push down on the inside of your knees with your elbows. Feel the stretch along the insides of your thighs. Hold for 10 to 15 seconds.

3. Repeat the stretch six to eight times.

Glutes Against the Wall

1. Lay on the floor, placing your body close enough to the wall that when your feet are placed on the wall, your lower back will be off the floor.

2. Place both feet on the wall, with one foot just below the knee of the opposite leg. This will stretch your glute area.

3. Switch feet and repeat the stretch.

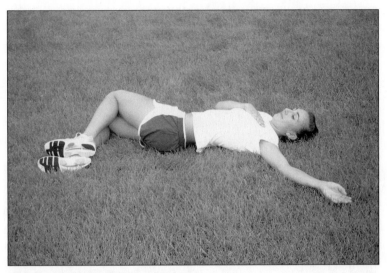

This Z stretch is good for the abdominals.

Abdominal Z Stretch

1. Using a mat or towel, lie on your back with your head flat against the floor.

2. Bend your knees, keeping your knees together and your feet flat on the floor.

3. Reach with your arms to the left side of your body; have your arms form a parallel line with your shoulders.

4. Drop both of your knees to the right side of your body (opposite your arms). Your body will resemble the letter Z. Hold for 8 to 10 seconds.

5. Repeat five to eight times.

6. Switch to the opposite sides, placing your arms to the right and your legs to the left. Hold 8 to 10 seconds.

7. Repeat five to eight times.

Waist Stretch

1. Stand up, utilizing straight posture, with your feet directly under your hips and your toes pointed forward.

2. Place your hands on your waist, with your elbows slightly bent, and then slowly raise both arms over your head.

3. Lean to one side until you can feel the stretch in your waist area. Hold for 8 to 10 seconds.

4. Repeat five to seven times.

5. Switch sides and repeat.

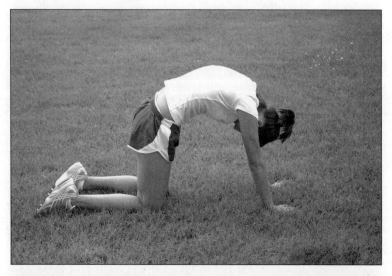

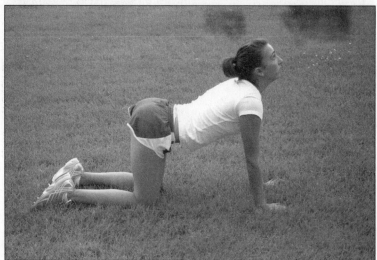

The cat stretch (left) and reverse cat (right) look simple and work very well.

Cat/Middle Back Stretch

1. Kneel and place your hands and knees on the floor.

2. Gently begin arching your back, rolling your shoulders forward and forming a "cat arch" with your back. You should feel the stretch in your back. Hold for 8 to 10 seconds.

3. Repeat five times.

Reverse Cat/Middle Back Stretch

1. Kneel down and place your hands and knees on the floor.

2. Gently begin swaying your back down, rolling your shoulders outward and forming a dip with your back. You should feel the stretch in your back. Hold for 8 to 10 seconds.

3. Repeat five times.

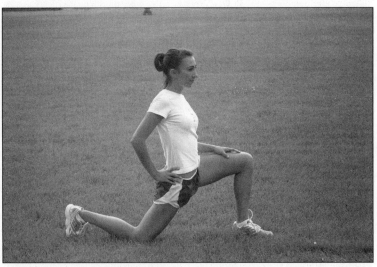

The hip flexors are another important area to stretch.

Hip Flexor Stretch

1. Stand with both feet together.

2. Step forward with one leg and bend all the way down in a lunge position. Allow the knee of your back leg to touch the floor and

move your hips forward. Keep your back and neck straight. Hold for 10 seconds.

3. Repeat three times.

4. Repeat with opposite leg.

Properly stretching the lower back prevents injuries.

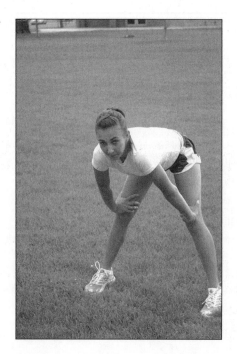

Lower Back Stretch

1. Lie on your back.

2. Slowly bring your knees up to your chest and wrap your arms around your legs.

3. Using your arms, bring your knees closer to your chest. Hold for 10 seconds.

4. Release; repeat five times.

An alternate version is doing one leg at a time. This will help loosen your lower back and spine area.

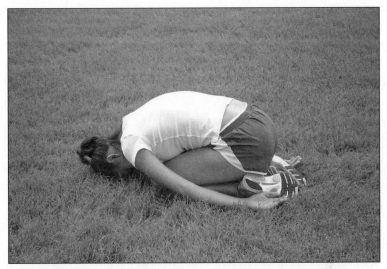

My team likes the "child" position stretch for the back and middle body.

Back Relaxation–Child Position

1. Sit on the floor, placing the shin area of your leg down.

2. Slowly bend your body down on top of your lower leg, curling yourself into a ball, as small as possible. Hold for six to eight seconds.

3. Repeat three times.

This is a great stretch to end your back and middle-body stretching routine, as it helps relax this muscle group.

Lower Body

From lunges to lower calf stretches, the following are great stretches for your lower body.

Lunge

1. Stand with your feet directly under your hips as wide as your shoulders.

2. Take a large step backward with one foot, creating a lunge position. Your body's posture should be straight, with your ears, shoulders, and hips forming a straight line.

3. Lean into your front leg; feel the stretch in your upper calf area. Hold for 8 to 10 seconds.

4. Repeat five to eight times.

5. Change legs and repeat.

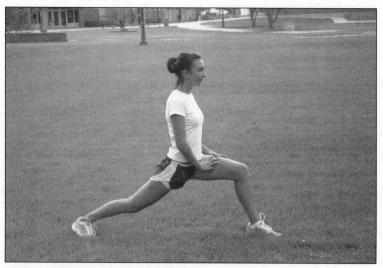

For targeting the upper calves, this lunge stretch is good.

Bent-Leg Hamstring Stretch

1. Sit with your leg straight and your other leg bent, with your foot at the knee of the opposite leg.

2. With your back straight and your head up, slowly lean forward at your waist. You should feel the stretch along the underside of your thigh. Hold for 10 to 15 seconds.

3. Repeat six to eight times.

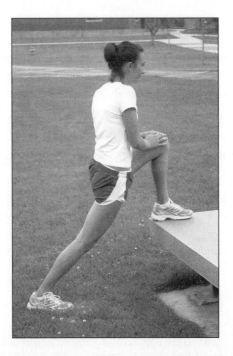

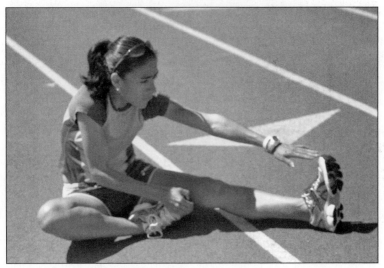

The hamstrings are a key, and these stretch that muscle.

Hamstring Rope/Belt Stretch

1. Lie on your back and wrap a belt or rope around your foot near the ball. Keep your leg with the belt on it straight and the other leg bent at the knee with your foot on the floor.

2. Slowly raise the leg with the belt toward the ceiling. Don't pull down with the belt; instead use your leg muscles to push up. You will feel the muscles along the back of your leg stretch.

3. Repeat twice.

Once you increase your flexibility, try this stretch, keeping the alternate leg flat on the floor. Repeat the stretch twice. Switch to the other leg and repeat the routine.

Hamstring/Bench Stretch

1. Stand facing a bench or chair and place your foot on the bench. It should form around a 75- to 90-degree angle with the floor.

2. Lean forward toward your toes until you feel the hamstring muscle begin to stretch. Hold for 8 to 10 seconds.

3. Repeat five times.

4. Switch legs and repeat.

Hamstring Stretch for the Mid-Rear Thigh

1. Lie on the floor with your back and head flat against the floor.

2. Bend both your knees and place both feet flat on the floor.

3. Extend one leg and maintain your leg approximately 2 inches off the floor with your toes pointed.

4. Slowly raise the extended leg toward the ceiling. Try to reach at least a 90-degree angle with your body with the extended leg. Hold for 8 to 10 seconds.

5. Repeat three to five times.

6. Change legs and repeat.

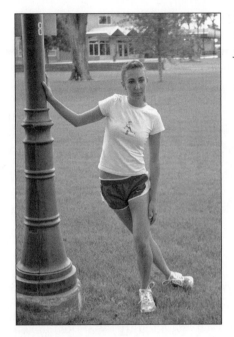

The IT band is a tough one to stretch, but this pose works fine.

Iliotibial (IT) Band Stretch

1. Sit with your leg bent and crossed over your straightened opposite leg, placing your foot near the knee of the opposite leg. Keep your other leg straight and flat on the floor.

2. Place the elbow of your opposite arm outside the leg with the bent knee. Slowly push your bent leg toward the opposite shoulder. You should feel the stretch along the side of your hip. Hold for 10 to 15 seconds.

3. Repeat six to eight times.

Quadriceps Stretch

1. Begin by standing along a rail or chair; stand straight with your leg bent.

2. Grasp the foot of your leg with your hand and slowly pull your heel to your buttocks. You should feel the stretch in the front of your thigh. Hold for 10 to 15 seconds.

3. Repeat six to eight times.

Upper Calf Stretch

1. Begin by standing near a wall and placing your hands on the wall. Put one foot behind the other.

2. With your leg straight, your heel flat on the floor, and your foot pointed straight ahead, lean slowly forward, bending the opposite leg. You should feel the stretch in the middle of your calf. Hold for 10 to 15 seconds.

3. Repeat six to eight times.

This exercise may be helpful for *Achilles tendonitis* and *plantar fasciitis*.

Lower Calf Stretch

1. Stand closer to the wall and bend one leg at the knee. Keep your foot flat on the floor.

2. Lean into the wall, which will intensify the stretch in your lower calf. You should not place pressure on the other foot.

3. Change legs and repeat.

Foot/Ankle Stretch

1. Begin this stretch by sitting on the floor with one leg lying flat and straight.

2. Bend the other leg in a 90-degree angle or to the point that your toes are pointing at the ceiling.

3. Grab your toes with your hands and pull back toward your body while keeping your leg in place. You should feel the stretch in your foot and ankle. Hold for 10 to 15 seconds.

4. Relax; repeat the stretch.

5. Change legs/foot and repeat the stretch.

Plantar Fascia Stretch

1. Place your hands on a wall and then place one foot on the wall; touch the toe to the wall. Your foot should form a 45-degree angle with the wall.

2. Lean into the wall with your upper body and hip area. You should feel the stretch both in the the bottom of your foot and the Achilles area. Hold for six to eight seconds.

3. Repeat three times.

The Least You Need to Know

◆ Stretching is as important as the workout itself.

◆ One of the best ways to prevent injuries is to have a smart stretching program. Not stretching causes and compounds injuries.

◆ A properly stretched body performs better. Stretching done incorrectly can derail your training plans.

Chapter 8

Your Strength Program

In This Chapter

- Why a strength-training routine can help you stay injury-free
- How developing key muscles keeps you on a healthy path
- What kind of strength training helps you—and what kind can hurt you
- Why a good strength-training workout should not take you even an hour

When most people think of running, they don't necessarily envision taut muscles and a six-pack stomach. When was the last time you saw a runner who looked like that? If you follow competitive running, you've more likely seen competitive runners who are lean, ropy, maybe even skinny. But don't be fooled: these lean, mean running machines are usually very strong for their body type.

Having strength doesn't mean bulking up, and this chapter isn't about weight training in the traditional sense. It's about bringing balance to your muscle groups and giving your comprehensive training program another tool to keep you not only fit, but also healthy.

Do It, but Don't Overdo It

Some runners don't believe strength training can benefit them, so they don't want to do it. Will a strength program really help you run better? You bet: it's been proven over time that runners who begin a strength-training program can improve their times. But there are better reasons than that, so let's get to it.

Your strength and weight training program should require at least a 10- to 12-week commitment. At Adams State, we look at strength and weight training as a year-round process, and we adjust the intensity and volume for the various phases of training. Anything less than 10 to 12 weeks won't provide you any real benefit, and could leave you sore and discouraged every time you start and stop.

Conversely, a lot of runners will jump into a strength or weight program with their regular intensity, then when they are so sore then next day they can't move, it's out the door. Don't overdo it right at the start. Don't get me wrong—you will get sore. But if you do it right, you can control the soreness and it will fade away, to be replaced with increased strength and fitness.

Dividing the Program into Phases

Developing an effective strength program means considering the entire picture before you begin. Divide your program into the base-building period, the precompetitive and competitive periods, and the postseason. Each of these will have a different focus as it relates to strength and weight training. The greatest amount of strength and weight work should be done in the base-building period.

Your greatest strength gains and greatest benefits will be realized in the preseason. During this base-building period, prioritize your specific areas that need work. Don't worry if you are just a beginning runner; a strength program works even better for a beginning runner. You won't usually be doing a lot of high-mileage work, so you can utilize your strength work more and realize the benefits as you progress.

As you move into the season, the precompetitive and competitive periods, you'll spend more time on your actual running and back off your strength program. The goal for this period is to maintain the strength you built in the preseason, lifting once or twice a week for each body part, typically one set of 8 to 10 or 12 repetitions. Be careful not to overdo it in season. Working hard on your running is the focus, and strength training is only an ancillary aspect.

During the postseason or transition phase, I recommend taking three or four weeks off from strength training. This allows your muscles and joints to rejuvenate for the next training phase. And when you do start back, start slow, with one set per body part once a week, working up to two and then three times a week, and two sets per body part. It is important to continue with a sequential, progressive program, and to do it consistently throughout the year.

Be Smart About Your Workout

As in all aspects of your comprehensive training program, be smart. Look over your plan and see where strength and weight training fits in for you. In this section, we will look at the various reasons to do a program and how it can translate into personal improvements.

A good strength program improves your muscles' ability to do higher-intensity training, such as hill running or interval training. The benefits of weight training are well known in the competitive running world. A complete and comprehensive program alone can improve a 10k time by over a minute. It aids in your body's ability to gain muscular strength and power input. Your muscles will be able to work harder and faster.

When you increase the strength of your muscles' connective tissue, you greatly reduce the risk of injury to muscles, connective tissue, and joints. Some common running injuries or running-related conditions can be avoided or moderated with a good strength program, such as runner's knee, improved posture, the ability to use your arms during training or racing, and many others. Too often your body is out of balance, meaning that the necessary complementary groups aren't balanced. Maybe your quads are strong, but your hamstrings are weak. This is an injury waiting to happen for most runners.

Consider your agonist muscles, a big muscle group that moves a joint around its access point, such as the quadriceps muscle that lifts the knee. An agonist muscle is also known as a prime mover muscle. When it is contracted, it is controlled and opposed by another muscle. The muscle it works in partnership with is called the antagonist muscle. The antagonist muscle slows or stops the movement of a joint and assists the agonist muscle in joint stability. The stronger those two muscles are, the more stable the joint is. This benefit will help when you do intensity training to increase your speeds, resulting in improved times *and* fewer injuries.

In Their Shoes

Amy joined our program as a tall, skinny distance runner out of high school. She is tall for a runner, around 5-foot-11, more like a basketball player, with very long arms and legs. This can be dream body type for distance runners, but not until everything is in balance.

Like a lot of skinny runners, she proved fairly weak in her nonrunning muscle groups and struggled with her form and biomechanics. But Amy was driven. Once it became clear that this was the main thing holding her back, she set herself on correcting it. She was a coach's dream! She didn't need any outside motivation from me—if anything, she needed me to hold her back a little.

Amy began a comprehensive training program, but we quickly found that a lifting program wasn't going to work for her. Amy's arm length and lack of upper-body strength didn't allow her to use traditional weights to build strength.

We decided to use her body weight as her resistance, and the clear path was established. Amy did sit-ups, push-ups, pull-ups, and many other resistance-type training exercises, using only the weight of her body as the tool. She began to build strength, which improved the way she carried her body, and ultimately made her a strong, contender athlete.

Amy went from the middle of the pack in high school to the top of the collegiate running world. In her senior year, she did what no other Adams State women's runner had done: she won three individual national championships, including the individual title; led our team to a national championship in cross-country, winning the 2-mile at the indoor national championships; and capped off her incredible year by winning the 5,000 meter at the outdoor national meet, establishing a new national meet record.

Amy is a wonderful example of what you can do when you set your mind to it. I always tell my athletes, it's not the body God gives you that matters; it's what you do with that body that will make you a winner.

As you put together your personal strength and training program, it's essential to understand what your body lacks and how to address it. I often suggest that if you're not completely sure, just work on each part of your body in turn, developing your overall strength as a place to start.

Begin with work on your arms and shoulders. In your arms, focus on activities that build both your biceps and triceps. For the shoulders, work on the deltoids located at the top of arm joint near the shoulder girdle.

As you build your lower body program, be sure to address not only the upper but the lower legs as well. Focus on the quadriceps and the hamstrings in the upper leg, and in the lower leg build the soleus (smaller calf) and gastrocnemius (larger calf) muscle groups.

One of the most neglected yet most important parts of the body is the *core*, the muscles in the stomach and lower back, and oblique abdominals on the side. This area cannot be overemphasized. It's the part of the body that holds you upright and connects all your extremities; if it's weak, it doesn't do a lot of good to have great legs and arms.

Runners who have weak cores show a lot of inconsistency in form and posture; they lean either too far forward or backward. When you have a weak core and start to tire, you find yourself leaning back. When you lean as your run, you can injure not only your back area, but your legs as well. Your legs compensate for the leaning, striking the ground out in front of your center of mass, creating a braking force that will over-fatigue your quads and possibly injure your shins.

Healthy Strength Training: How It Adds Up

Strength training is comprised of three different components. The muscular component deals with the muscle's ability to hypertrophy (become larger), apply force, and shorten and lengthen. When we talk about lifting for runners, we don't want the muscle to become large; we just want to strengthen it.

The neural component involves the brain's way of sending messages to the muscles and receiving information back, affecting how the muscle reacts. Strength training provides stimulus in the brain that works to control frequency. As the frequency increases, the message exchange

Watch Your Step

Large muscles tend to produce heat, so it's important for performance reasons to strengthen the muscle without it becoming too large. This will become more important as we talk about the kind of lifting to do. It's also why we want to lift lighter weight for higher repetitions rather than heavy weights for lower reps, which builds bigger muscles.

has to happen faster and faster. As more muscle is used, more tissue is recruited and activated. All of these together train your body to react quicker and get more benefit for faster muscle building.

The mechanical component deals with the angle of the joint and range of motion of the joint. To get the most from your joints, you should be working to improve your range of motion. As these areas become bigger and smaller, it has an effect on how you lift and build strength.

Different Approaches to Strength and Power

There are many different approaches to building strength and power: calisthenics, machines, free weights, medicine balls, and so on.

Isometrics involves exerting force on immovable objects such as a wall, so you're not lifting, but rather pressing against or pulling on something. There's no movement of the joint, so there is no range of motion. You can create varying loads as part of the workout, and I suggest two to three sets. This type of program has not been proven to be as effective as other types of strength and lifting for athletes. After around five to six weeks, the benefit of isometric work diminishes, so you'll need to move to another phase to fully benefit from the strength training.

For variety in your strength training, try circuit training. This system is effective, but it can be complex. You will need to have between 10 and 20 work stations, each with specific exercises. You begin at one station, complete the activity there, and then move onto the next station for the next one. You could have a dumbbell curl be one station and push-ups be another. Another work station might be a medicine ball drill and another some type of calisthenics.

Another key type of strength training is dynamic weight training, which includes lengthening and shortening the muscles through the movement of the joint. There are basically three different types of dynamic exercises. Isotonic exercises involve the use of free weights throughout a full range of motion. This is best applicable to sports and athletics. This type of work allows you to transfer more of the strength it builds into useful activities.

Watch Your Step

In my college program, I am a big believer in medicine balls. They come in all different weights ranging from 1 kilogram all the way up to 10 kilograms. These ball activities help improve your range of motion and they can be used in throwing exercises to develop strength and power.

Isokinetic exercises provide constant resistance, generally done on the resistance or hydraulic machines you find in health clubs or gyms. As you apply force to the machine, it in turn applies an equal and opposite force back to you throughout the full range of motions. So the load changes or varies as you work with/against the machine during the workout.

The third type of dynamic training is balance. Muscle groups that work together need to be balanced with the coordinating muscle group. Most athletes can relate to the one involving quads and hamstrings. When one of these muscles is considerably stronger than the other, an injury can occur. They don't have to be equal (that's almost impossible), but there is a strength ratio that allows the muscle to work the best and limits potential injury. We generally use quadriceps at 60 percent strength and hamstrings at 40 percent, so a 60/40 quadriceps to hamstring ratio is fairly good. Once that ratio moves to around 70/30, your risk of injury is greater. Having muscles that work together or in opposition be in balance is our goal.

Beware the Overload

I would like to share a few concepts related to the law of overload. As we begin to do more lifting, more weight, repetitions, and more sets, the law of overload allows the body to adapt, but only if we give it time to adapt. So we increase the volume and intensity to allow our body to "stress" in a healthy way to promote adaptation to occur.

When we work these muscles, we have to incorporate activities that use a full range of motion. If we start out using too much weight, we will only be capable of a limited range of motion and won't develop the whole muscle. Using a full range on all exercises also prevents certain imbalances that lead to injuries.

It's vital that you allow proper time for recovery. When we engage in a strength-training program, it takes a certain amount of time to recover from it. It could take 48 to 72 hours or even longer for a specific area to fully recover from a hard strength workout. Space out your training sessions to allow this needed recovery time. I suggest something like a Monday/Thursday or a Tuesday/Saturday program.

Making Your Own Program

I suggest you personalize a plan for yourself and make regular changes to eliminate any boredom, thus keeping the program new and fresh. You can find additional exercises and activities that will meet your personal interests and needs in a multitude of resources.

You should be able to do your whole workout in about 30 to 40 minutes. And if you do a circuit workout and move quickly from station to station, you could complete the workout in 20 to 30 minutes because you're bringing a cardiovascular aspect into your workout.

As you implement any strength or weight program, be sure that you fully understand the activities and take precaution to complete them safely. A part of that safety program is to learn and understand how to breathe when you lift. There are distinctive breathing patterns that make lifting more comfortable and safer.

For example, if you are doing the bench press or a push-up, when your arms are fully extended, your chest should be contracted, and as the bar or bodyweight is brought down—called the "negative" motion—you inhale a breath in and the chest expands. You bring the negative down in a two count, and then as you push the bar or your body weight up, you exhale as you continually push the weight to where the arms are locked out. The pushing motion is in a one count and the lowering of the weight is in a two count, so the lowering takes twice as long. As you learn the different activities, pay careful attention to when and how to breathe.

Exercises for Strength

In this section, I am going to share a variety of exercises that you could incorporate into a strength program. Remember, you can use any of these exercises, all of them, or none of them. You can combine weight training with machines and exercises that only use your body weight. Find a program that works for you and that you enjoy, so "working out" doesn't become just "hard work." They are not intended to be all-inclusive, nor do I think you should perform them all each time.

Front Leg Raise

1. Lie down with your upper body supported on your elbows; keep the knee bent on the alternate leg.

2. Flex the top thigh muscle. Hold for a count of three to four, then raise your leg and hold for an additional three to four seconds.

3. Complete two or three sets of 8 to 10 repetitions.

Side Straight-Leg Raise

1. Lie on your side, placing your hand on the ground in front of you near your body.

2. Flex the thigh muscle of your top leg, and then slowly raise the leg off the floor. Hold your leg in this position for three to five seconds.

3. Complete two to three sets with 8 to 10 repetitions in each set.

4. Repeat using the alternate leg.

Straight-Leg Raise

1. Lie on your side with the alternate leg crossed over the knee.

2. Place your foot on the floor directly in front of the knee of your remaining straight leg.

3. Lift the straight leg; hold for four to six seconds.

4. Do two to three sets of 8 to 10 repetitions.

5. Change sides and repeat the process.

Wall Strength

1. Stand with your back against the wall and your feet 6 to 8 inches away from the wall.

2. Slowly lower your body until you're in a sitting position, pushing back against the wall. Hold this position for 8 to 10 seconds. You should feel your thighs begin to tighten.

3. Stand up; repeat 8 to 10 times.

All you need is a wall for this one.

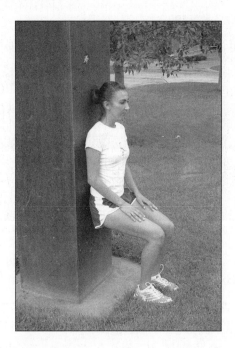

Stomach Straight-Leg Raises

1. Lie flat on your stomach.

2. Tighten your thigh muscles and slowly raise your leg about 1 foot off the floor. Hold this position for four to six seconds.

3. Do two to three sets of 8 to 10 repetitions.

4. Change legs and repeat.

Superman Exercise

1. Lie on your stomach.

2. Lift your arms and legs high into the air. You will feel your stomach stretch. Hold for 8 to 10 seconds.

3. Repeat three to five times.

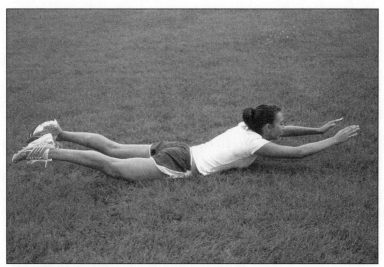

The Superman exercise strengthens lower back and stomach muscles.

Arm Curls

1. Using a barbell or a can of soup, curl your arm up, moving your arm from a hanging position until your arm touches your bicep.

2. Repeat the curl 10 times, and do two to three sets.

3. Change arms and repeat.

Dips

1. Standing beside a chair or bench, place your hands on the bench, holding up your body weight with your arms. Hold for 8 to 10 seconds.

2. Repeat three to five sets.

3. Progress to dipping down with your body, much like doing a push-up, supporting your body as it moves alongside the bench.

Squats

1. Stand up, with your feet shoulder width apart and your knees directly over your feet.

2. Lift your arms up and cross them on your chest.

3. Squat down and then return to standing.

4. Repeat eight times.

5. Another variation is to not cross your arms, but instead hold a lifting bar across your shoulders and repeat the exercise.

Calf Raises

1. Stand on the edge of a step or stair using only your toes and forefoot for balance.

2. Rotate up and down, moving your foot both above and below the step.

3. Repeat for two sets of 8 to 10 repetitions.

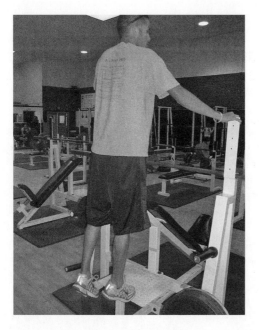

These are great for strength-ening your calves.

Working with Your Body Weight

Weight training can be an asset to your program. However, I would also encourage you, whether you have access to a gym or not, to work out on your own.

To do that, you use the best "weight" around: your own weight. Doing push-ups and pull-ups, squats without weights, and lunges with your body weight are good for both flexibility and to build strength and endurance. Working with your own body weight also keeps you aware of just how much you weigh and what kind of shape you are in. As you work out, starting with push-ups or pull-ups, you will see that in time you're able to do more repetitions or more sets. This is because you're not only building strength but also losing weight—or at least decreasing your fat percentage and increasing your lean body mass.

Herschel Walker, a noted sprinter and former NFL football player and U.S. bobsled team member, maintains he never worked with weights, instead doing crunch-ups, push-ups, and other activities with only his body weight. Yet he had a chiseled frame—and still does into his 40s. The good part about push-ups, sit-ups, lunges, and squatting is you can do them anywhere, even (and especially) at home, with no equipment.

A pair of light dumbbells might also be a good investment, because you can use the dumbbells to raise the level of effort in squats and lunges. You can also add arm curls and arm extensions for the biceps and triceps, respectively, and some shoulder raises and presses, along with some one-armed rows.

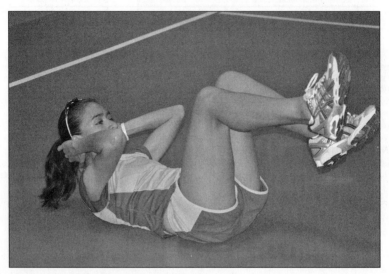

Doing crunches and sit-ups builds core strength.

The Least You Need to Know

◆ Don't use heavy weights and fewer repetitions, because it builds too much mass.

◆ Find a workout that keeps you motivated and does not take a lot of time.

◆ If you do not have a gym, you can still work out at home, with or without weights.

◆ Like with any other aspect of training, when working out, listen to your body.

◆ Doing calisthenics, push-ups, and pull-ups—working with your body weight—is a great way to get fit.

9

R & R: Two Important Letters

In This Chapter

- ◆ Why the body needs some time off
- ◆ How to step back even when you're improving
- ◆ How to train yourself to relax
- ◆ Why sleep helps you avoid common sicknesses

I am not a very good sleeper—never have been. Even when I was training myself, I found it difficult to commit to the correct amount of sleep. My coaches would tell me and I somehow knew it was helpful, but I could never seem to sleep the full amount I needed. Only when I began to train athletes did I realize what a disservice I was doing not only to myself, but to my potential.

No Rest Equals No Recovery and No Improvement

When I entered the coaching profession and began to study the effects of training, I learned very quickly how important good sleep patterns can be to your overall health and fitness. Telling a group of college students to get a good night's sleep and to commit to rest is certainly a challenge, but those athletes who want to succeed and understand the complete system of training will do it. And as other athletes see the accomplishments of those runners who commit to health and training as a lifestyle, they, too, tend to join in.

When I teach students or train elite athletes, I make sure they know that recovery is as important as workouts. Without a good and full recovery, your body doesn't function well. Continued training without adequate rest will lead straight to injury and illness.

The Bad Effects of No Sleep

So you think it's impossible to set aside 9 to 10 hours per day to sleep while you're training hard? You can't quit your job to sleep, so with all your other obligations, you think it just can't be done.

If you are one of the many people walking around today without enough sleep, it can cost you plenty. The quality of your work as well as the quantity is negatively impacted when you are sleep deprived. Your ability to concentrate is decreased and your coping skills are lessened. The lack of proper sleep can have a major negative impact on your training and can quickly lead to injury or illness.

Let's just consider one of the obvious types of injuries, the one where you just weren't functioning at full mental capacity and made a dumb mistake. This type can occur in the blink of an eye, and an injury such as a nasty fall messes up your training for several weeks.

When you don't sleep enough, you tend to decrease the amount of time it takes before you are exhausted when doing aerobic exercise. This lessens your training effectiveness and keeps you from completing workouts at the level you desire. While your body is impaired by the lack of sleep, you are sending a decreased amount of energy to your muscles, too. This will create unneeded and unproductive stress on your system and reduce your running efficiencies, resulting in a lower performance than you would have accomplished if you had only changed your resting patterns.

Watch Your Step

The Korean national marathon team has used Alamosa (and the surrounding area) as a training base a couple times during my tenure. We seem to have an ideal training environment for marathon training. We've had national teams from Korea, Italy, Japan, and Tanzania, as well as individuals from all over the world, come here to train.

The Korean team focused on high-mileage running and preventing injuries, running three times a day five to six days a week.

When they didn't run three times a day, they would go for one long run. On a couple occasions, their coach would drive them out to the Great Sand Dunes National Park and have them run all the way back, a route that took them nearly 38 miles. The entire route is somewhat flat and straight, and these runners ran at close to a 6:10/mile pace for the entire run, finishing in less than four hours. I truly wouldn't have believed it if I hadn't seen it with my own eyes. Once this workout was complete, they stretched for an extended period, then used ice, massage, and other recovery methods.

And then they would sleep. Sleeping 9 to 10 hours or more at night did not suffice, as they would have one or two afternoon naps as well. All in all they slept as many hours as they were awake.

This is an example of what it takes to run successfully in a high-mileage training program. The sheer volume of mileage they ran required a tremendous amount of attention to recovery—and an emphasis on rest to achieve that recovery.

This type of running can work for some, but more often than not it is not sustainable, as the risk of injury is high. But on the two occasions that this group trained in Alamosa, I never saw one of their athletes injured to the point that he couldn't run. I truly believe that their rest and nutrition allowed them to maintain this training regimen without suffering severe injuries.

Another side effect from not sleeping enough is the body's decreased immunity to illness. Ever notice that when you are feeling run down and fatigued, a cold or flu bug is right in your path? Lack of adequate rest and sleep make you susceptible to even the smallest types of illness.

And once you get them, they are even harder to get rid of if you don't commit the time necessary for rest and recovery.

Polypeptides—Follow the Z's to Complete Recovery

Have you ever awoken from a night's sleep, maybe even one that lasted seven or eight hours, and felt like you didn't sleep at all? You may feel groggy or just lethargic, not your usual perky, first-thing-in-the-morning self. This probably means you didn't complete all the necessary cycles of sleep to cleanse your body of the waste it produces. Without the adequate amount and/or cycles of sleep, you are left feeling sluggish.

Sleep is probably the most underutilized area of recovery, and probably the most important. We each need different amounts of sleep to reach our potential, and research shows that as a general population we don't sleep enough. I would bet that most of you don't get nearly the amount of sleep you need to maximize your training and feel your best.

REM: It's How You Spell Sleep

If you are training hard, you need nine to nine-and-a-half hours of sleep per night. With that amount of sleep, you'll get about three hours of REM (rapid eye movement), during which your body will remove chemicals from your blood, including polypeptides, which accumulate while you are awake.

As you rest, your body removes polypeptides. Your body uses your cycles of sleep to cleanse away the polypeptides. However, this cleansing only truly takes place during REM sleep. That's why it's so important to sleep long enough to have at least two and possibly even three phases of REM sleep.

When you sleep long enough to complete the different sleep cycles, you allow your body to feel more refreshed and you wake up ready to attack your workout more aggressively.

The Keys to Getting Enough Sleep

Are you one of those people who would sleep more if you could? You're not alone. Many people find themselves watching the clock all night, stressing about the fact that they want to sleep but can't. You might expect that running, especially running hard, should help you. But many runners find themselves still looking for ways to get more sleep and get the most out of it.

Evidence suggests that increasing your amount of exercise does improve your ability to sleep. But for those of who are sleep challenged, that exercise needs to be several hours before bedtime. Exercise stimulates your metabolism, which is your goal, but it also keeps you from relaxing and sleeping until several hours have passed. So if you suffer from an inability to fall asleep, adjust your workout time to morning or lunchtime. Allow yourself a few hours to wind down before bedtime. Runners who do this fall asleep quicker and experience longer and better sleep.

Another key to getting to sleep and staying asleep is limiting your intake of caffeine. I have noticed that some runners still feel the effects of that strong coffee up to 12 hours later. If you aren't sleeping well, stop drinking caffeine after lunch and see if that helps. Also, keep in mind that tea, soda, lattés, and even some energy bars have caffeine as well. And stay away from energy drinks, the definition of high caffeine.

Pay attention to when and what you eat as your bedtime approaches. If you eat your evening meal too late, your body is still digesting food and during that working process, it isn't as easy to get to sleep. Also, if you are prone to indigestion or reflux, stay away from spicy foods near the day's end.

Set a schedule and stick to it. Establish a waking hour and a sleeping hour that you can stick to as close as possible. Over time, this type of routine will train your body to sleep and wake up just like clockwork. Your body know when it needs to be awake and be ready when it's time to sleep. The more regular you establish your training, eating, and sleeping habits, the better your body will respond.

Take a look at your sleep environment. It's no wonder that hotels across the country are adjusting to a new spalike atmosphere for their rooms—it works. A comfortable bed, good mattress, and the right pillow make entering the sleep zone a pleasure. It also helps if you can control the light and temperature in the room. A slightly cool, dark room is ideal for that needed rest.

Overtraining to the Point of Sleeplessness

If you find that you have eliminated all the barriers to sleep but still have difficulty resting, consider whether you are overtraining. If you are, your body will have great difficulty recovering from workouts. Another sign or symptom of overtraining is an increased heart rate when you wake up each day.

Napping can feel great when you're training hard, and I certainly enjoy a short doze in the recliner after a hard workout, but it doesn't help keep your sleeping patterns at their best. Most naps don't last long enough to do your body much good in the recovery phase—they mostly just interfere with the good night's sleep you'll need. While napping works for some, I don't recommend it as a way to address the issue of getting enough sleep. More often than not, napping will interrupt your daily routine and prevent you from getting that much-needed good night's sleep.

Another indicator of overtraining is persistent soreness and stiffness in your muscles and tissues. This soreness can sometimes be felt in your joints and tendons as well. Loss of appetite is another warning sign that you may be training too much and not allowing your body to rest and recover.

If overtraining could be contributing to your inability to sleep and recover, back off. You may be able to improve your sleeping experience just by easing up on the intensity of your workouts without adjusting the mileage. If adjusting the intensity doesn't help, lower your mileage until you can get the rest and recovery component of your program under control.

The Coin's Other Side: Relaxation

In our world today, we run both literally and figuratively every day. If you're lucky, most of your running involves shoes and a nice trail. But all too often our running is in our everyday activities, chores, and even in our work. It's no wonder that relaxation is way down the priority list every day.

But relaxation is vital to good overall health and an essential part of the cycle of training and improving. Without it, your body will reach a stress point that brings on all types of minor illnesses and can contribute to the overall failure of your training goals. Don't let an inability to relax and recover be a hindrance to your training and/or racing goals.

Sitting down in your favorite chair and letting your body go limp isn't usually the hard part. Learning to relax psychologically is a very important part of recovery as well. A lot of runners become obsessed. You may have a personality type that is very driven, and running is an activity that can become very addictive as you get into it. If you tend to overwork yourself in other areas of your life, pay extra attention to the need for relaxation and your process for letting your body and mind relax and recover.

Watch Your Step _____

Some of the overlooked benefits to relaxation are how it impacts the response your body creates to stress, such as ...

◆ Lowering your blood pressure.

◆ Slowing your heart rate.

◆ Increasing the flow of blood to your muscles.

◆ Reducing muscle tightness or tension.

◆ Assisting in slowing your breathing rate.

There are major overall health and wellness benefits to relaxation activities. Athletes who practice these techniques tend to have fewer physical stress symptoms such as headaches and/or back or neck pain. Relaxation helps you deal with your emotions from a higher level of awareness, cuts down on negative emotions such as anger and frustration, and gives you added patience for everyday problems and negative situations.

Relaxation techniques use activities and mental skills to help you refocus your attention to something calming and increase awareness of your body. Try different ones or even combinations of techniques until you find the ones that give you the relief you're looking for. Often the technique for relaxation before sleeping will be different from the one you use to calm before a race or big event.

Visualization Helps You See Success

Visualization uses the mental process of refocusing your attention off the random thoughts or stressful activities at hand to a calm, serene place or situation that enables you to let down.

Try thinking about something peaceful. I find it helpful to work my way through a journey in my mind. Quietly and calmly think of a calm, peaceful place and begin moving yourself into this place in your mind. Use all your senses. What does it smell like? What can you hear? Often my peaceful place is a shaded and wooded area near the ocean. Think of the cool breeze and the soft sound the water makes. Feel the warmth of the sun on your skin and then imagine how the sand pushes against your feet. Spend a few minutes completely relaxed in your ideal place, and then slowly bring yourself back to your current state.

Internal Relaxation

This technique uses a combination of body awareness and visual imagery to help you relax and reduce stress. Think of words or phrases that help you move out of your current stressed state and into a relaxed mode. Combine these thoughts with a conscious activity that relaxes your body, such as slowing your breathing rate. Take several long, slow breaths, exhaling thoroughly. Think of yourself floating in a cool pool of water on a warm day. Think of the refreshing splash of water that cools you down and refreshes your senses. Take one extremity at a time; relax the muscles first in each leg, then in each arm. Continue by tensing then relaxing the muscles in your body, neck, face, and head.

Progressive Muscle Relaxation

This one is probably my favorite and the one that I suggest most often when asked about a relaxation technique that helps get you into a calm and serene environment. This technique alternates between muscle tension and then muscle relaxation, enabling you to learn the different sensations. You'll learn to identify the times when your muscles are tensing and focus on relaxing them before the tension spreads and gets you too uptight.

Read through the entire exercise before beginning. It is important to understand the different points where you need to pause. Adjust the pause periods for the optimum length of time to help you achieve your goals. Sometimes runners tape the instructions and add in the pause periods so that they can listen to the tape and not have the distraction of reading the instructions. After doing the exercise several times, you'll learn the different phases of relaxation and can do the process by visualizing it in your mind.

You should be wearing comfortable, loose-fitting clothes and no shoes. Sit or recline into a comfortable position. Close your eyes and tune into your own breathing patterns. *Pause.* Notice the rhythm and pace of your breathing. *Pause.* Take another breath, a little deeper this time. *Pause.* Take another breath, again a little deeper; let yourself feel completely calm and peaceful. Think of yourself in a quiet, comfortable, and relaxed state. *Pause.*

Breathe in slow and easy. Take several breaths. *Pause.* Begin by clenching your right fist. Squeeze tighter and tighter. Clench it as hard as you can. Study how the tension is building in your fist, then building in your hand, then building in your forearm. *Pause.* Release, relax. Now let your fist and hand relax and go limp. Allow each finger to hang loosely. *Pause.* Notice how different you feel when you clench your fist versus when your hand and fingers are hanging loosely and completely relaxed. *Pause. Pause again.*

Relax your whole body. Let go and relax even more completely from your head to your toes. *Pause.* Bend both of your arms at the elbow, and begin to tense your biceps. Keep building up the tension in your biceps until they feel rock hard. Hold them tight and feel the tension. Study how the tension feels in your arms. *Pause.* Slowly and easily let your arms go back to a straight position. Gently drop your arms down to your sides. Go limp; relax. Notice how your arms feel heavy when they are relaxed. Be aware as the tension leaves your muscles and you begin to relax the tension in each muscle of your body. Spread that feeling into the rest of your body. Seek a feeling of peacefulness and calm into your body. Notice how you are beginning to feel more and more relaxed. *Pause. Pause again.*

Now move your focus to your neck and shoulders. Tense the muscles in your upper back and follow that by tensing your shoulder and neck. *Pause.* Begin to relax; breathe in deep and easy. Let the muscles in your upper back, neck, and shoulders completely unwind. Let them down when you relax. Think of the tension leaving your neck and shoulders and notice how heavy the relaxed muscles are. As you release and relax the muscles in your arms, neck, upper back, and shoulders, notice how relaxed your upper body area feels. Your torso and stomach are now relaxed and the tension in your lower back area is easing as well. *Pause.*

Move to the lower half of your body. Tighten and flex the muscles in your buttocks and thighs. *Pause.* You can increase the tightness in your thighs by pressing down on your heels while keeping your toes in the air. *Pause.* Hold the tension. *Pause.* Keep those muscles tight. *Pause.* Now let go. *Pause.* Relax your hips, butt, and thigh. *Pause.* Allow the feeling to spread into your legs and upper body. Think of the relaxation process and how your upper body is loose and relaxed now.

Begin by pressing your toes away from your body, much like you would if you were standing on your tiptoes. Work until you feel the muscles in your calves tighten up. Pull your toes up and back toward your shins. This will work the calves and increase the tension. *Pause.* Hold the tension in your calves. *Pause.* Relax and release. Let the tension flow right out of your legs and the relaxation flow down to your toes. *Pause.* While you are completely relaxed and loose, breathe deeply and slowly exhale. Repeat these breathing techniques three or four times. Slowly return to breathing at a normal rate.

As you end your relaxation state, take a deep breathe, wiggle your toes, shake your legs, shake your arms, roll your head around on your neck, and open your eyes. You will feel relaxed, refreshed, and calm.

Time Off Whether You Need It or Not

In early June, I send out training programs for the college athletes I work with to follow over the summer. When they return in August, we really get things going and train hard until our racing begins in mid-September. At that point, we are in full-swing cross-country mode until the national meet in late November. This is a long time for young athletes to train hard without a break, so when the season ends, it's time to stop, rest, and regroup before moving into indoor track later in the winter.

Do you need to take time off? Even if you're not following a strenuous training or racing regimen and are just staying fit and focusing on good health, you do need some time off after several consecutive months of training. Once you've run several (if not every) days a week for a few months (five or six is my suggestion), take a transition period to let your body rest and revitalize.

During training phases, your body uses its stores of vitamins and minerals and can approach depletion. Your muscles and joints get impacted every day when you train, and giving them some time off helps them return to normal before you start the process again. A rest period of one to two weeks gives you a chance to heal and regenerate naturally. If you train over several months in preparation for a big road race or possibly a marathon, it's even more important to take time off and adjust your body back to an easy phase before you continue on your training path.

Another key part of taking a transition period is mental. I have seen runners who do too much for too long and get "runner's burnout," a dangerous phase for even the most die-hard runners. If you reach the point that running is no longer fun and more of a chore than a pleasure, you may find yourself wanting to hang up the shoes for good. Before you reach this state of mind, give yourself some time off. When you come back to running, you'll have your old excitement and enthusiasm.

If you're too stressed about your fitness level to take a complete break, consider some low-impact or moderate cross-training activities. Walking is a great alternative to running during the rest phase and still gets you outdoors and enjoying the scenery in your community.

When you return to running, start at about 50 percent of your highest volume before you began the rest cycle. Gradually increase your training time until you reach an adequate level of time/distance for your overall fitness and conditioning. Once you have been back at it for four to six weeks or more, add back some hard workouts or that local road race for a change of pace. Keep in mind that you won't set a personal best, but you'll be rested and ready for a little harder work. If you want to race for true competition, wait until you have returned to your full training mileage before toeing the line.

I want to caution you, time off is important in your overall health and fitness plan. It will benefit you both mentally and physically. But don't let yourself get too far away. If you go too long without hitting the road, you could find yourself starting completely over in your fitness and training programs. Take the needed time off, but get back out on the road and run as soon as you are recovered; you'll be glad you did.

The Least You Need to Know

◆ A good night's sleep is as important as training and eating right.

◆ If you are overtraining, it can cause restlessness at night.

◆ No matter what, you need to take time off.

◆ Your mind needs a rest as much as your body.

3

Running and Dressing Defensively

You may think you're ready to run, but first we have to get you in the right shoe. It's essential to get the right equipment on your feet, and that's what shoes are. We are also going to spend some time looking at gadgets and apparel, and even talk about some treadmill running.

Okay, then—it's snowing out. Or it's 110 degrees. Should you run? Let's consider the elements and what kind of running surface you head out on. These are important factors if you are to stay injury-free. We also talk about the running environment in general, especially pesky cars and potentially dangerous animals.

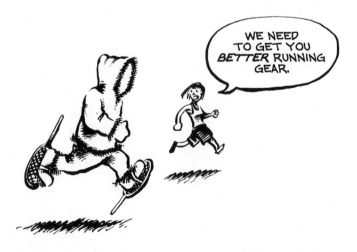

Chapter 10

If (and Only If) the Shoe Fits

In This Chapter

- ◆ How to figure out your foot
- ◆ How your stride affects the shoe you need
- ◆ The best way to analyze your shoe needs
- ◆ How to best care for your running shoes
- ◆ What to ask a shoe salesperson when you're shopping

You won't make a more important running-equipment purchase than your shoes. The retail landscape is littered with bargain shoes—though sometimes there's a reason those fancy-looking "running shoes" are only 10 bucks and are sitting in the clearance bin.

Running shoes come in as many different shapes and sizes as the human foot. If your foot rolls inward when you land as you run, you don't want a pair of shoes built to compensate for a foot that rolls to the outside. So to prevent injury and to properly spend your hard-earned dollars—this is, after all, an investment in yourself—we're going to look at how what you put on your feet has a lot to do with injury-free running.

Shoes: The Most Important Purchase

Fall is an exciting time around the small town of Alamosa, Colorado. The college students return and, for a small town whose population increases by 20 percent during the annual student influx, you can just feel the excitement in the air. The student athletes who run for our college team bring added excitement to our community. You see, our town views the local cross-country team the way most places get excited about their football or basketball teams.

We kick off the return to school with a time trial to see which athletes did their homework over the summer. I also use it to determine who will make the traveling competition team and who will be transitioned to the developmental program. I hold a special place in my heart for the entire incoming freshman class; unlike the upperclassman, they have no idea about the incredible ride they are about to begin.

I know a great deal about each of the athletes who join our program. They give me regular updates on their training and send me results from their high school competitions and any road races they run. But one year, I had several new young women runners who I was very anxious to see compete in the time trail, so I could better understand where they stood in terms of fitness.

We arrived in front of the school early on Saturday morning. Runners new and old were warming up and getting ready to go. As the newcomers toed the line, I looked down and couldn't believe my eyes. One of the freshman girls was wearing combat boots! She came from a very poor family; they didn't have the resources to buy the right shoes or equipment, so she ran in army boots. But she finished the time trail surprisingly well, considering her shoes.

I didn't say anything to her that day, but I was sure that everyone noticed, and I'm sure she also understood how lacking her equipment was. I scheduled an appointment with her for early Monday morning to figure out a way to get her the right shoes. And what a difference the new shoes made! Her times continued to improve and, as the season transpired, she eventually made the team, competing at the conference and regional meets as a true freshman. What a lesson she taught us all with her perseverance.

Running is a simple sport. You go out the door and put one foot in front of other. You don't need a court, pads, or even a scoreboard to be a successful runner—but you do need good shoes. You wouldn't show up to play baseball without a glove, so don't consider lacing up for a run without the right shoes. It's an equipment decision that will affect your ability to stay healthy more than any other.

Anatomy of the Shoe

Venture into a local sporting goods store and you will be awestruck by the multitude of shoes. They usually divide them by sport, but occasionally you will just see a wall of shoes. They come in a million colors; some have a unique shape or maybe just a new logo. The reality is that shoe styles are cyclical just like clothes. Often manufacturers will phase out a style or color and replace it with the newest, greatest design and color.

Granted, there *are* new and occasionally major breakthroughs in shoe design and construction, but not as often as every season. To help you sort through the different types of shoes, let's look at the different parts of the shoe and the role they play as you run.

The upper portion of the shoe is generally lightweight and in some models can actually have air holes for ventilation. These holes are great for circulating air in the heat, but can freeze your foot off if you are running in the cold.

The bottom of the shoe, called the *outsole,* is the part of the shoe that strikes the ground. You need it to be durable and give you the proper traction for the training you plan to do and the surface you plan to run on. The tread will be for straight-ahead motion, unlike cross-trainers, which have tread that goes from side to side.

The liner of the shoe is referred to as the *insole.* It is generally removable and provides an added layer of support and cushion. Note the height of the arch support inside the shoe; it will need to match your own arch design. (More on that coming up.) Supination occurs when your ankle rolls out, so that your weight lands more on the sides of your foot

This is an example of supination.

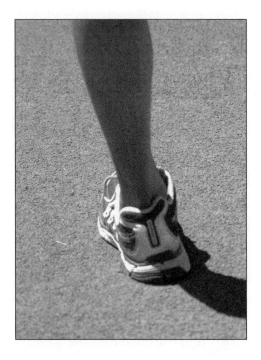

I consider the key area of the running shoe to be the *midsole,* the area directly above the outsole that provides most of the cushioning. This is often done using air pockets or gel. One of my personal favorites is the dual-density foam. I find that this combination of foam provides both support and cushioning. This section of the shoe is the equivalent to a shock absorber, and just like in a car, you need to find the one that fits you the best.

The last major section of the shoe is the heel counter area. Located on the back around the heel, it is usually the strongest and most sturdy section of the shoe. You want something with a firm heel so you have a solid base and your foot doesn't move around.

The size of the toe box is also important. Not all toe boxes are created equal, and you will need to be sensitive to the one that matches your toe size. You don't want one that is too large, or your toes will move too much. But you don't want one that is too small, or your toes will be under pressure, and in no time you will have blisters or black toenail.

A shoe's flexibility needs to match how your foot works. A good test is to pick up the shoe and fold it. Does it bend where your foot does—in the front section of your foot, not the middle where your arch is located? Flexibility is important in keeping plantar fasciitis or Achilles problems to a minimum.

Your Golden Arches—Treat Them as Such

Motion control shoes provide stability features to help control motion on the medial side (middle part of your foot near the arch). To find the right shoe for yourself, you will need to do a complete assessment of your foot and your biomechanics. Assessing your foot will tell you the type of shoe you need before you ever try on a pair.

First look at what kind of arch you have. Begin by wetting your foot and then stepping onto a piece of construction paper or cardboard. Your foot will leave a simple impression where the wet area touched the paper. That's the area of the foot that is supporting your weight. As you run, those are the areas that are going to take the most stress from running. Do this for the other foot, and then take a pencil and trace the outline so that you can look at it later or take the drawing with you to the shoe store.

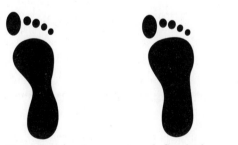

Examples of arch types: normal, flat, high.

Normal Arch

There are three types of arches: normal, flat, and high. A normal arch has a distinct curve along the inside of the foot with a band a little less than half the width of your foot connecting the heel and toe. You generally have normal pronation. Pronation is the medical term that refers to the rolling-in or flattening out of the foot's arch, which can result in flat feet.

With a normal arch, your feet and ankles are strong enough to support your body and you tend to have good control when you run. Runners with this kind of arch will normally see the forefoot area (the balls of their feet), their toes, about half of the outside of the middle of the foot, and then the entire heel on the paper.

If this is you, you can basically wear any kind of shoe. You want to select a shoe that matches your running motion; this is a good foot for running, so you don't need a shoe with all the bells and whistles that control the motion of the foot.

Flat/Low Arch

If you have this type of foot, you won't see much of a curve through the middle part of your foot. It can look like your foot is full from heel to toe. You will notice that where the arch is will be a wider wet impression—thus a flat foot. Typically this means that you *overpronate*— that your heel and ankle can't support your entire body weight.

Overpronators often have a larger and or heavier body type. This can be from weight issues or from a larger body frame. If you fall into this category, you will need more cushioning and firm support. Runners with low arches deal with stability and motion-control issues.

An example of pronation.

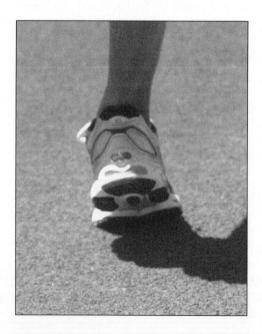

When shopping for shoes, look for dual-density midsoles and supportive posts on the outside of the shoe to help control the motion when you run. This type of shoe will also lessen the oscillation of the foot. As your foot strikes the ground, you have a somewhat inward roll and tend to push off the front part of your foot (forefoot). You may find yourself pushing off of your big toe, which can present a risk of injury. Look for a shoe that will allow you to push off with three or four of your toes and not just the big toe.

In Their Shoes

It's all in the shoes. Or is it? Rick was a walk-on athlete from a small town in northeast Colorado. He joined the Adams State men's program, and everyone wondered if he had a chance. Rick didn't begin the season keeping up with the front-runners, but the coaches began to notice some interesting things about Rick. When we took his heart rate after intervals, it returned to normal much quicker than you normally see with athletes at his level. We soon realized that his body was truly designed for hard running.

Rick trained hard and found himself on the national travel team. One benefit that year's team received was several pairs of shoes; like most of the team, Rick packed them up and hauled them to nationals.

As he lined up in the cold, frigid weather in Wisconsin, Rick was focused. As the race began, it soon became clear that this young sophomore was about to break out from the pack. He took the lead a little past the 1-mile mark and controlled the field. This was something that many of us never get a chance to see.

Rick neared the finish line well ahead and enjoyed the final stretch. As the remaining runners finished and the team victory became apparent, the celebration began. When Rick sat down to change into his cooldown apparel, one of his teammates looked down and asked, "Did you wear those shoes on purpose?" Rick had worn two different shoes: one was a spike and the other a flat. Rick replied that he hadn't noticed, before or during the race! It goes to show that the mind is stronger than the feet when it comes to racing.

High Arch

With this type of foot, you will see a very sharp curve along the inside of your foot, and the wet imprint of your middle foot will show a much thinner band. This type of foot normally belongs to *supinators*, or underpronators.

When your foot is shaped like this, you basically do not have the oscillation of the foot going inward as you strike your heel and the foot comes forward; you tend to roll on the outside edge of your foot and push off with your little toe. Runners who have a very high arch have an increased risk of injury if they don't have the right shoes. Your weight is not distributed evenly over your foot compared to other types of feet.

If you are in this category, I suggest that you look for shoes that use a neutral control. This type of shoe does not guide your foot either in or out; it allows it to remain neutral, so you don't supinate or pronate. These shoe types encourage your foot to pronate and help you distribute the shock of landing on your foot. You won't need a stability post, as having one will exacerbate the problem of underpronation of the foot.

Selecting What's Right for You

As you assess your personal foot characteristics, it will be important to know what you want from each of the different sections of you running shoe. Always remember, you are looking for a running shoe—not a jumping shoe or a walking shoe. Shoes built for running are different from other types of athletic shoes and are designed to support you when you put one foot in front of the other day in and day out.

Running shoes come in three basic shapes. Some models are built with a curve in them. This model will look like the arch is carved in or cut away. A model with a lesser curve is designed so that the forefoot points slightly in on the shoe. A straight model is a shoe with an arch area that looks almost straight from top to bottom.

If you have a normal arch and pronate normally, you can select from a wide variety of basic training shoes. Look for shoes with good flexibility, an adequate amount of cushioning, a semicurved shape, and no medial post.

Runners with a low arch or flat foot who overpronate should search for a shoe with good motion control that will assist your foot from rolling too far as your run. They generally have a straight shape; a medial post that extends to the arch; and a strong, thick midsole—this will give your foot maximum support. They are generally the heaviest shoes on the market and provide control-type support.

And last, if you are a runner with a high arch and supinate, look for a shoe with great cushioning. This type of shoe will support your foot as you roll inward while you run. A curved shape with a soft midsole will be your best bet.

How Will You Use the Shoe?

If you are a beginner, then you will need a basic running shoe. It should fit your foot correctly and give you the needed support. As you advance in your running program, you may find yourself interested in what I call specialty running shoes, made for different running situations such as racing or hill or off-track training.

Shoes designed for racing situations are much lighter and don't have the needed cushioning and support that you will need for longer distances or training day in and day out. Don't be fooled into selecting them because they look pretty and feel light—they are truly made for racing only.

Shoes for trail running have additional stability built in to give added support to your ankles and knees when you run on terrain that is unstable or unpredictable. They tend to be a little wider and slightly heaver than the basic training model.

The Ultimate Feat: Shoe Shopping

As you begin your quest for the perfect shoe, I suggest looking for a sports store that specializes in running shoes and apparel. These types of stores often have runners working in them who will immediately know how to answer your questions and fit you with the right shoes.

If you find yourself in a store with a wide variety of shoe types, don't settle for the first salesman that comes up. Instead ask some questions and find the right salesman who knows running and running shoes. A good shoe salesman will do some shoe tests, such as the water on paper test, on you. Sometimes he or she will ask you to walk around or even put you on a treadmill to watch your running form. These are all good techniques to help decide which shoe is best for you.

Watch Your Step

Some factors to consider when purchasing shoes are:

◆ Your level of running experience, from beginner to long-timer.

◆ Your running goals—are you training for a marathon or just trying to lose some weight?

◆ Your current and projected mileage.

◆ The main surface types where you train.

◆ Any foot issues (arch type, weight, toes, blisters).

Plan to spend 30 to 40 minutes looking for a pair of shoes. Take your time on this and don't be in a hurry. When you are trying shoes on, it's important to bring the pair of running socks you will wear with you. If you have to borrow socks at the store, make sure they are similar to the ones you will wear in terms of thickness. This will give you a better indication of how your foot will feel inside the shoe when you get home and start running.

Put the shoe on and maybe run up and down the sidewalk outside a few times. If there is even a little issue with your foot feeling too tight or your toe pushing inward, the shoe is not going to feel better when you take it home and start to run with it—it's going to feel worse, and you will need to find another pair.

I like to try on several pairs of shoes and see which one feels better and why. Narrow it down to two pairs, and put one shoe on each foot and jog a little bit or walk and see how each feels. Then switch shoes. If you do all that, you'll avoid a lot of problems.

There might be cases where you like the shoes, but they feel too narrow or loose. Several companies make shoes that have different width. Do try on several widths to make sure you get the right pair.

The Point of No Return(s)

Another good thing to ask the salesperson is the store's return policy. A lot of good running shoe stores will usually allow you to return it for a new pair as long as you don't abuse the shoe and return it quickly. Keep this in mind as you develop a relationship with them, because you will likely be buying more shoes from them if things go well.

Many times good training shoes will cost roughly between $60 to $150 or even $200. I think you can get a very good shoe for $75 to $90. When you find the right pair, buy them, and if you really love them after trying them out for a while, buy a couple more pairs—before the manufacturer moves on to something else.

Avoid the marketing campaigns, and forget how cool or pretty the shoes are. You want a shoe that suits your foot, your running style, and your training plan. Pay homage to your needs, and don't get caught up in the bright colors and new stripes.

Shopping online can be a great convenience, but I suggest doing this only after you have purchased and worn a particular shoe and know that it works for you. Nothing can take the place of trying on your shoes and having a professional help you determine the fit.

Some people like to compare shoes to tires on a car, but they are actually a lot more than that: your shoes are your shock absorber and sometimes your steering wheel, and it has to deal with proper alignment.

Shoe Care

A running shoe will usually last about 350 to 500 miles. It depends on how many miles you run a week; it could be as little as a couple of months for someone in a high-mileage program, but for a novice it could be six months. Looking at the total mileage is important—even though the outside of the shoe and top doesn't look worn, or even the tread, the foam rubber or EVA Foam inside the shoe can be compressed over time. That foam loses its ability to expand and contract and eventually becomes compacted. That can make the running surface you are running on harder, even though the shoe looks fine from the outside. So pay attention to the mileage you put on the shoe.

Taking good care of shoes is important. One of the most common mistakes is washing shoes, which can damage them the most. You don't want your shoes to look bad, but washing them can break down that foam in a hurry. And once you have damaged the gel or foam, you've damaged the entire shoe. Putting them in the dryer is a huge no-no because it will harden the rubber and foam and make it more dense. The shoe won't cushion the blow of striking the ground. If you have to clean them, use a little soap and a wet cloth on the outside, but never under any circumstances put them in a dryer.

> **Watch Your Step**
>
> Once you put a certain amount of miles on your shoes, the best thing you can do is throw them in the trash. A lot of athletes want to keep the shoes. But wearing shoes that are broken down will actually hurt the runner by altering biomechanics. Wearing broken-down shoes even for everyday walking can damage your feet and make your legs and back hurt.

I encourage my runners to purchase two pairs of shoes. When you go out for a run and put miles on them, you compact the rubber inside of them, and it takes time for the rubber to expand and go back to its normal shape and size. If you run in the same pair of shoes every single time, the process happens even faster and the compacting worsens. If runners alternate shoes, this allows the shoes to last longer and gives them time to recover and be in good shape. You will be wearing a better shoe if you have two pairs.

Enjoy getting the right shoe! It will be your friend as you train and will do more than anything else to keep you on the path to injury-free running.

The Least You Need to Know

+ It's important to get shoes that have arch support if you have high arches.

+ Select shoes that don't rub or have any uncomfortable pressure spots. Shoes that don't fit right when you buy them will never fit right.

+ Take the kind of socks you will run in with you to buy shoes.

+ Spend as much time as needed trying on shoes, walking and jogging with them before you purchase.

+ Feet come as different as shoes—make sure yours are a perfect fit.

Chapter 11

Apparel and Equipment

In This Chapter

- ◆ How to shop for running clothes
- ◆ Building a weather wardrobe
- ◆ Gadgets and gizmos

Shopping for running gear and gizmos is a very important part of injury-free running, because wearing the right gear prevents injuries and illness and keeps your focus where it should be—on putting one foot in front of the other.

The electronic accessories you might need range from monitors to a treadmill, but let's talk about why and when you need these in this chapter so that you save money and make the right purchase for the right reason—as in, if you need it, let's get it.

Not Just Off the Rack

What should you wear? As you consider your best bets for running healthy and injury-free, you still want to look and feel great. The following information gives you some perspective on the types of choices you have that will prevent injuries related to climate and still protect your body against everything from rashes to blisters. Let's start at the beginning—where the skin meets the fabric.

Underwear

Select undergarments that fit you snugly and protect your skin from chafing. Fabric type is key; select a soft yet comfortable product and not only will you look good, you will have the layered support you need for a great training session.

Sports Bras

The most important purchase in running gear may depend on if you are a man or a woman. I generally place shoes as number one, but lots of women runners I know would argue with that—to them, a good sports bra makes all the difference.

Purchasing a bra that fits correctly seems to be a challenge in the regular world of undergarments. Adding the needs of a sports bra makes it even more complicated. I suggest going to a store specializing in running and/or sporting gear. Try on as many as you can; it really is the best way to see which one will work for you.

Watch Your Step

If you are large busted, you are looking for a style that will give you the fit you need and the support you want. Try the bra on, bend over, jump up and down, do a few stretches—does it stay in place? Lean over; you shouldn't move too much or fall out over the top. Does it provide the containment you want? If you are small busted, you are looking for containment and coverage. Put the bra on and look in a mirror; does it cover the way you want it to?

The bra should fit comfortably around your body, with straps that adjust and provide needed support. The fabric should be soft and comfortable to prevent chafing and thick enough that it holds your breasts close to your body as you run. Consider the closure types that will work best for you: over the head, back snaps, or a front zipper—each has pros and cons, but it is all about the one that you will enjoy wearing.

I suggest fabric that is easy to launder and won't shrink or stretch. Ask the questions you need, get professional help if available, and go with the one that works the best for you.

Running Socks

Running socks can prove to be a valuable investment when running long distances. They wick away moisture and help prevent those nasty blisters that runners often get. The best fabric for running socks is generally a blend. Do not wear 100 percent cotton socks; they absorb moisture and can cause your feet to develop blisters.

Runner Facts

Most running socks are made of a lightweight blend that contains at least two moisture-wicking materials that work together to prevent blisters. The layers help absorb friction between layers and move moisture away from your feet. As the moisture gets to the outside layer, it evaporates, so your feet stay dryer.

Consider your climate and running environment as you select socks and in all your workout plans. Running on trails or uneven surfaces requires a sock with a little support, but during interval training or repetition running, a thinner sock helps. The weather and/or season can affect the fabrics you require as well.

Insoles Keep You in Step

The most important fit you can get in running is your shoes. Ideally if the shoe fits correctly, then you won't need anything extra to help prevent injuries. But for some runners an insole can provide some assistance.

If you need a little added oomph in your shoes, I suggest an insole that provides cushioning. Over-the-counter types work great; just select one that fits your foot and your shoe properly. Remember—if your shoes are worn out, adding an insole won't help and could make you more injury prone.

The other insole type provides stability. These are generally a little harder and have a molded arch support added. This type of insole can aid you if you are inclined to pronate as your run. Often runners with plantar fasciitis problems will find some relief when adding a supportive insole in their shoe.

Dress for (Running) Success

Most runners turn compulsive when shopping for racing gear. Whether you're looking for shoes or your racing outfit, you will likely be looking for something lightweight that keeps you cool. Racing outfits can vary quite a bit depending on your taste. Some runners prefer that the outfit fit a little tighter than training gear.

Racing shorts have an optional split leg that gives you a little more freedom of motion while you run. Most importantly, pick something comfortable and fun. Racing is generally the highlight of months of training.

Success in Layers

The secret to staying comfortable in varying temperatures is to layer your clothes. How many layers and what fabrics you use depend on the season and moisture conditions. The market for running attire has lots of options to choose from; just know your needs before you spend.

I suggest you comprise your running wardrobe of several different components. If you're running in hot or humid weather, select a fabric that wicks moisture away from your body as your perspire. It will keep you more comfortable and prevent that heavy, yucky feeling that you get from a soaked cotton T-shirt.

If you're running in the cold, then select undergarments that are made from fabrics that keep your body warm, while removing moisture that tends to make you feel colder. Layering is key in cold climates, and your outer layer serves an invaluable role.

There are multiple products that aid in climate control; each is great when it comes to keeping you dry and warm. It wasn't that many years ago that when it rained, you would be soaked from head to foot. But today, with products like Gore-Tex, you can stay much more comfortable and dry. Indeed, there are materials for just about every running situation. Besides the normal fabrics—cotton, nylon, and tri-cot—you can now choose Gore–Tex, Polartec, Climacool, or Coolmax, not to mention Supplex, Tactel, Dri-Fit, and Lycra. With so many choices, you're bound to find the perfect fabric.

It's common knowledge that tights can keep you warmer on a cold, wintry day. Manufacturers have now developed a Lycra-based compression fabric that claims to reduce soreness. This particular tight will fit snugly and provide greater muscle support.

Give Yourself a Hand (Cover)

When it's cold, wearing gloves is a must. Keeping your hands and fingers warm keeps the blood flowing and keeps your focus on the workout in front of you. For days when there is just a nip in the air, I suggest a light pair of gloves that allows the skin to breathe and not become too warm for comfort.

As the temperature drops, you need hardier coverage. Several different glove types will meet this need. Select a warm pair made from a fabric that provides wicking to remove moisture from your skin.

Watch Your Step

Your throat and mouth can get really dry in the cold air; remember to drink water as needed.

Several types have an outer mitten shell that protects from moisture and can also be pulled back when your hands become warm. An interesting yet valuable feature is the sweatband that some gloves contain. It is useful for removing sweat or whatever else might be dripping as you run on cold days.

In Their Shoes

Zoila Gomez loves the marathon. As a college athlete, she won six national titles in distances ranging from the mile to the 10k. As she moved from college competition to running as a professional athlete, the marathon became her favorite race.

Zoila is a budding star in the marathon circuit, finishing third in the United States marathon championships as well as having a great debut marathon in New York earlier in the year. She now finds herself in the wonderful position of racing on behalf of the United States in the world championships in Osaka, Japan.

As Zoila and I worked on her racing strategy and training plan for this incredible event, it became obvious that the heat in Japan in mid-September would be a factor. To prepare for these conditions, we researched and concluded that a hydration strategy would be our primary focus. Zoila plans to take in between 4 and 6 ounces of liquid every 15 minutes during the race.

Preparing to run a world championship marathon is difficult; adding the component of training for a hot marathon in the cool weather of Alamosa, Colorado, makes it that much harder. In order to be ready, Zoila has been wearing one or two layers of tights while running in the hottest part of the day. This will help her begin acclimating to the heat stress of the actual race. We also have planned to train in Houston, Texas, for two weeks before she finishes her final two weeks preparing in Osaka.

As we studied how to implement that type of hydration strategy, an interesting tidbit came out. When you run in a hot and humid climate, not only will your feet sweat on the inside of your shoes, but drinking as you run will result in water dripping on your shoes, as well as sweat dripping down your legs and off your arms onto your shoes. We discovered that if you spray your shoes with Scotchguard before you run, it will help repel the water and keep it from soaking through to your foot. Keeping your feet dry will help prevent blisters. It is equally as important to protect your feet from the inside as well. Zoila picked a poly/cotton lightweight sock manufactured to wick away moisture from the feet.

Sunglasses

Sunglasses are a valuable and important asset when you train. They help block out harmful rays from the sun, prevent you from squinting and straining, protect your eyes from bugs, and help aid your vision to watch for hazards while you're running. It's important to find the right pair for you and your running environment.

When buying sunglasses for running, make sure they provide adequate safety and protection for your eyes. Your sunglasses must give you 100 percent UV protection.

There are many problems associated with not wearing sunglasses with proper protection, including problems such as cataracts and macular degeneration. A big misconception is these troubles only affect adults. Runners of all ages, including children, should wear UV protection sunglasses.

All sunglasses have some UV protection, but not all sunglasses present the same UV safeguards. You should look for sunglasses that offer the best protection you can afford. Polarized lenses are a great option as long as they have adequate UV protection. These lenses will cut down on glare created by the sun. Wrap-around sunglasses offer outstanding protection, because they block peripheral UV rays from the side. Sunglasses with light-tinted lenses will not block out the glare of the sun.

Select frames that fit comfortably; many are too tight and create discomfort after wearing them even a short time. After deciding on the type of sunglasses you like that also offer the protection you want, your choice should come down to which provides you the most comfort.

It seems that every model of sunglasses provides several options of colored lens tints, and many models now have interchangeable lenses. Just make sure that all the interchangeable lenses offer 100 percent UV protection. When selecting a color lens tint, you should consider when and where you plan to wear your sunglasses. A dark lens (brown/amber) would suit runners who are running in bright areas or near large bodies of water. A lighter lens (yellow) can increase clarity in low-lighted areas and are great for running on shaded paths.

Runner Facts

Everyone has unique features that will need to be addressed while purchasing sunglasses. Remember that most sunglass manufacturers make different sizes of the same sunglasses, or offer similar models with different sizes.

Caps and Hats

Protecting your head and face from the sun is the primary purpose of caps. When the heat is on, select a lightweight cap that wicks away moisture from your head. A terry headband can provide some relief from sweat getting into your eyes as well.

Road Blocks

Always keep your head covered and pay special attention to your ears. The outer edges of the ears are easy targets for frostbite, often in just one cold morning run. You will find yourself miserable if you fail to protect your ears.

During the cold weather, hats are vital. Skull caps are popular, and there are many types to choose from. Some come with optional ear flaps, and most are made of fabric blends that keep the heat in, yet pull the moisture away from your head. Keep in mind the size of the hat and check for good coverage before making a purchase.

Reflective Apparel

The best option to stay injury-free is to run in the daylight, but if you must run when light is scarce, at least be seen. Long winters bring short daylight hours in many parts of the country and leave lots of running enthusiasts in the dark.

Watch Your Step

Wear sunscreen and/ or a moisture cream with sunscreen for winter running. The cold air can chap your skin very quickly.

If you find yourself running either before or after the sunlight hours, be sure to wear reflective apparel. There are several different jacket or vest options, but all will help keep you safe from the traffic.

Treadmill Training

Sometimes the weather just won't cooperate, and the risk of injury is increased by the conditions that Mother Nature hands us. During those times, I recommend getting in your workout on a treadmill. Consider your climate and your budget, but if owning a treadmill is in your plans, here are a few things to consider.

Treadmills protect you from the elements, but their own environment is fairly boring. Models that provide programmability are helpful in addressing this issue. Look for ones that can simulate different courses to provide some variety. Incline adjustment is essential, and be sure your treadmill can do this with the push of a button and does not require manual adjustment.

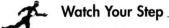

Watch Your Step

At the very least, the treadmill should display your time, pace, distance covered, and speed. Often models can give your heart rate and calorie burn. These are great motivators when an inside workout becomes a little boring.

The motor is key; get one with at least 1.5 horsepower. You don't need one strong enough to power the group at the local health club, but you don't want to feel like the treadmill can't keep up. It should be able to go at least 10 mph, or about a six-minute mile pace. If you plan to do workouts faster than this (and your fitness supports it), you will need one that go up to 12 mph.

Consider your size and the frequency you will be working out on the treadmill when making a selection. If you are a larger runner, be sure the model you select can handle the pounding that you will provide. Having a model that's too slow or too fragile will keep you from using it the way you should. Find a vendor that will let you try one out. It's the best way to know if a treadmill is the one for you.

There are some safety tips to remember while using the treadmill. Be sure to have some air circulation in the room. Point a fan in your direction. This will prevent some sweat and keep it off the belt, which can create a hazard. Always use the emergency stop feature—it's there to protect you during a fall. And don't forget—warming up and cooling down are just as important on a treadmill as they are out on the road.

Jogging Strollers

With all the competing demands for time, it seems that few of us have time for running. If we have young children, we may need to also take the kids for a ride. To do so without injury can be a challenge, but jog strollers have made it easier.

Pushing an additional 30 to 50 pounds can present a hazard to your back and legs. Using a jog stroller that has large, 20-inch rear wheels works best. A safety feature that assists in injury prevention is a front wheel that locks in a forward position when running and then unlocks when you are maneuvering sidewalks and doorways. Look for a model that has an easy-to-use hand brake. Try to find one that folds easily, as this will come in handy when storing it.

Accessories

You can spend as much money as you want on various running gadgets and accessories. Some of it is stuff you need to monitor your efficient workout—and some of it just makes your running experience more enjoyable.

Watch My Time

One of the most basic gadgets runners need to help them train correctly is a good watch. Good doesn't mean expensive; it just has to do a few fundamental functions. When I look to purchase a watch, I want one that is simple to use and one that I can see from an arm's length when I look down. I think the face size and the readability of the time are the number-one considerations.

Runner Facts

As you select the level of memory capability that you need, consider how often you will do sessions that require lap/split recording, then factor in how often you will retrieve the information from your watch. Generally a watch that records around 50 laps/splits will meet most runners' needs.

Having memory capability that matches with your workout sessions will make the training experience go better. Watches have capabilities that range from as few as 10 laps to well over 100. Most of today's models allow you to store that information so you can add it into a running log later. Memory-recall mode needs to be easy to understand and simple to use, otherwise a week of workouts will be known only to your watch.

Like most other electronic devices, watches have evolved over time to include just about anything and everything. Some measure altitudes, have alarms, convert time zones around the world, and so forth. I recommend you get one that does the functions you will use and not much more. Pushing the wrong button and seeing the time in Tokyo is no help during a speed workout session.

Plug In to Stay Tuned In—to Your Body

As you move through the various phases of training, knowing your heart rate can be a key factor in your development. Runners at different stages of training and experience can either overwork or underwork during running and not even know it. When this occurs, not only will you not get the results you're after, but in the event you are training at a rate that exceeds your target range, you can injure yourself.

A heart-rate monitor can be a great tool. I recommend getting one that uses a chest strap with a sensor and a transmitter (often a watch). This style tends to be the most accurate and easiest to use.

Frills are everywhere, and you can add as many different options as you desire. Some higher-end models gather and store information over the course of several workouts and allow you to download this information to your computer. Of course, this type can be more costly, but it does allow you to track and even graph your heart rate over time, which can assist you in analyzing your workouts. If you don't select one with a computer download option, pay close attention to the memory capability. It is important to have enough memory to capture data from multiple workouts for comparison purposes.

Other options include models that calculate calorie expenditures, altitude measurement, and VO2 Max measurements. When you are considering the models that require sending signal (from the chest sensors to the watch), make sure they have a coded signal. If they don't, you could find yourself experiencing interference caused by other runners who are wearing heart monitors, too.

Portable Entertainment and Headphones

It seems that many of us need a little music in the background while we run. There are many models of music players on the market today (and improvements happening all the time) that will accomplish this goal.

In the spirit of injury prevention, let me just say that you should pick something small and light, and look for cords and headphones that won't create a tripping hazard. Many new models have great headphones that stay put regardless of how fast and furious you are working out—but they do prevent you from hearing some of your surroundings. Be careful and stay attuned to the environment, and recognize that you aren't always hearing the danger around you.

Key Storage

Yes, this really does have to do with injury-free running, because trying to stash your key in your shoe or sock is an injury waiting to happen, and jamming a key or keys into your waistband can cause skin irritation or even puncture injuries, wounds exacerbated by sweat and dirt.

Over the years, I have seen every type of storage plan for runners. Everything from straps around the arm to keys tied to shoes. While lots of these options work, they can sometimes cause unintended injury should you fall.

I suggest a small pouch that fits between your shoe laces and provides a cushion between you and the keys. It's very important to never store items (keys, money, and so on) inside your shoes—that's a major blister waiting to happen.

Hydration Packs

Keeping hydrated during a long run is essential to good health and injury prevention. During our long training runs, we provide water at multiple points during the workout, but when you're training on your own, I suggest developing a hydration plan.

This can involve planned stops during your workout where you know that water will be available or taking water along as you run. A very simple option is the water bottle designed to be carried by hand. This option works for runners who don't mind having an object in their hand as they run.

If that doesn't suit you, then a hydration belt is the next step up. Several models carry varying amounts of water and come with options that range from a key holder to pouches that hold your jacket and enough space for a picnic lunch. I suggest a compact model that provides you with enough water for your average long run and fits snugly around your body to prevent chafing and overheating as you run.

For the more sophisticated types, hydration packs that use a bladder and a tube that goes right into your mouth are available. These units are designed for running situations that require you to stay focused on the terrain, or you might just prefer not using a traditional water-bottle-type system.

All of these options work; it really depends on your personal preference when selecting a hydration system. What isn't optional is staying hydrated as you train.

The Least You Need to Know

◆ Match fabric to the climate in which you run.

◆ Your ears are very vulnerable when you run in freezing temperatures.

◆ Ask questions when buying sunglasses. Function is important.

◆ If you're a larger runner, don't pick a tiny treadmill with a narrow belt.

◆ All hydration options have benefits. Pick the one that works for you.

Chapter 12

Weather and Where You Run

In This Chapter

- ◆ The safest pavement for your knees
- ◆ Why grass is and isn't a good running surface for injuries
- ◆ When training on a running track is appropriate
- ◆ How to deal with the coldest weather
- ◆ The best way to handle the heat
- ◆ How to combat shifts in temperature

It's time to head out for an afternoon run, and you're wondering which route to take. If you're lucky, you will have many options and be able to vary your training utilizing multiple surfaces. Variety will not only cut down on the boredom factor, it will assist you in staying healthy and injury-free.

However, you often don't have lots of surface choices for running workouts; or maybe you have become a creature of habit and you only go one way every day. Here's some information on making good choices about the different types of surfaces available.

Cementing the Truth

Let me begin by pointing out the absolute worst surface that you can run on: concrete. It's generally made up of cement, another term for crushed rock, and has virtually no give. It hands your body a shock every time you run on it and can be a major contributor to shin splints and stress fractures.

I know city runners are cringing right now, and I will completely acknowledge that concrete can give you an even and consistent surface to run on; however, the pounding that your body takes over the long haul will make you more susceptible to injury.

Asphalt

Only slightly better than concrete, asphalt has a little more give and can be gentler on the legs. Asphalt is probably the most common training surface for runners and is often the fastest and easiest one to access. It's generally predictable and sturdy. Most road races are, well, on the road, so most runners do at least some of their training on the roads.

But asphalt is made of a mixture of gravel, tar, and crushed rock, so it's still a hard surface. Also, asphalt is poured on streets at an angle to help drain water, so if you are running at the side of the road, you'll notice a slope that can knock your biomechanics out of whack and lead to serious injury if you don't alternate the angle at which you run.

I would caution you to limit your training time on asphalt as much as you can. It's unforgiving and can cause the same type of stress injuries on the legs as concrete. Another key reason to avoid asphalt is that it's designed for cars—not a good mix for runners from a completely different injury perspective.

Treadmill

Treadmills provide a predictable and even training surface for your runs. They come with a variety of features that allow you to adjust everything from how many hills you intend to conquer to the speed and resistance you are craving that day. Setting the machine for the various paces is limited only by your ability to keep up. There are as many models as your imagination can process, and you can spend as much or as little money as you want. Additional features include calorie counters, heart-rate monitors, and even built-in fans and entertainment systems.

The big drawback of treadmills is that they limit any environmental variety and can be become boring very fast. If you drift off, so to speak, as you work out, you may find yourself flat on the floor with treadmill belt burns. Because of the lack of wind or fresh air, be prepared for excessive sweating.

However, treadmills play an important role in injury prevention by providing an alternative to runners who don't have access to acceptable training surfaces or who live in climates that aren't conducive to outdoor training.

Tracks

Running on a track can be great fun for short periods, and tracks are truly ideal for speed training or interval workouts. Most tracks today are made of synthetic materials and provide a medium-hard surface. Occasionally you can locate an old cinder track; they will generally be a little harder than the synthetic surfaces.

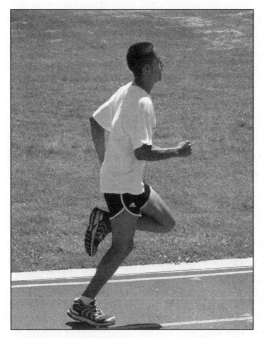

Running track surfaces are getting better.

All the elements that make a track great for intervals—400 meters around with two curves and two straight-aways—also can make it boring for any other type of training. Repetitive trips around the track in the same direction (another one of those runner's habits) can be hard on the knees and hips. To get the most out of a track and stay injury-free, use it for intervals and speed, not for your long run on Sunday.

Sand: When Running's a Real Beach

Being located near the Great Sand Dunes National Park gives me the chance to experience running on sand from a unique perspective. The sand is a mixture of wet or dry flat sand and some fairly incredible sand dunes (hills).

Running on packed, wet sand can be a good, soft surface as long it's level. I am not a big fan of running on dry, loose sand. It can give your legs an incredible workout, but the potential for injury may not be worth the gain.

> **Watch Your Step** _____
>
> Carry identification with you everywhere. Should you get hurt or have any sort of medical emergency, you want a Good Samaritan or emergency personnel to know who you are and how they can help you. If you have any type of medical condition, be sure to note that as well. A good spot for putting this info is on the sole of your running shoe or in a pocket on your running shorts.

The most common place runners encounter sand is at the beach. While you can sometimes find wet, flat sand on the beach, there is the potential for injury if the sand is too slanted or too loose and deep. If you're looking for variety, run on the sand as the exception and not the rule.

Sling Blades of Grass

Runners are always looking for a nice grass field, where the grass is short and well kept and the ground is smooth, level, and even. Unfortunately, golfers don't generally like to share.

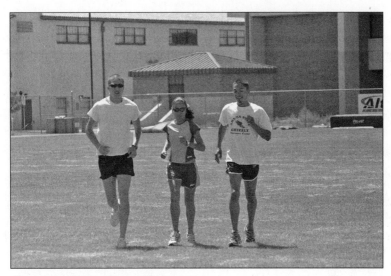

Grass is good—but dangers lurk.

If you can find the right spot, grass is a great surface to run on. It provides a good cushion and gives your muscles a quality workout as well. It lends support to runners who might be recovering from a stress fracture, and if you feel an ache or pain coming on, it can be a great alternative to harder surfaces.

Grass is king, but it can still have hazards. Watch for holes and uneven areas hiding under taller grass. Sometimes grass will cover water and you won't know it until you are sliding along. Unstable grass terrain is not for runners prone to ankle injuries. Also keep in mind that those with allergies may have a great run today and then not be able to breathe tomorrow.

Hitting the Dusty Trail—Which Might Hit You Back

I would say that trails designed for running are your best friend. Trails can come in a variety of surfaces and generally keep you away from traffic and other hazards. Trails made of dirt are easier on your legs and can prevent overuse injuries. They reduce impact on your legs on the downhill as well.

Be aware, though, that conditions on dirt trails can change quickly. One downpour and you can go from ideal to injury. Always watch for wet and slippery spots, and if you're lucky enough to have a dirt trail that winds through the trees, watch for roots and branches, too.

Trails made from woodchips rank as my number-one running surface. If you are fortunate enough to live in or near a community that has developed these types of trails, be sure to take advantage of them. They offer a medium to soft surface, generally on level ground. They are away from cars and can go on for miles and miles.

Variety is your best bet for injury-free running. Whenever possible, find surfaces that are medium and absorb shock rather than deliver it. Try different routes, look for parks, or find your local track. Running injury-free is something you can do almost anywhere.

Weather or Naught: Bad-Weather Training

I have lived in the high-altitude desert environment of Colorado for over 20 years. At around 7,600 feet, we get some incredible weather: the summers are made up of warm days and cool nights, and the sun shines almost 350 days per year. However, here in Alamosa we also have the distinction of sometimes being the coldest spot in the nation. While the humidity is low (thank goodness), the cold and wind are very real.

I approach weather as just another variable in our training program. My athletes sometimes cringe when they hear me say "It's a beautiful day to run," on the coldest, snowiest days. But staying injury-free as we strive toward our training goals is always my intention.

Cold-Weather Training: Running in Layers

Winter weather is no reason to stop running—or to even stop running outside. With some commonsense approaches to dressing and safety, you can go all winter and never miss a day! In fact, I find winter training days to be some of the most enjoyable.

Always Be Visible

Winter gives us a lot less sunshine to enjoy and brighten our path. Getting out there and soaking some up really helps with our moods and spirits.

It would be ideal if you could train or work out during the warmest, brightest part of the day (even if it is only 10 degrees), but most of us in the real world can't adjust our schedules to accommodate this.

If you must train in the early morning or evening, be sure to wear reflective gear and bright colors, and choose a lighted path.

> **Watch Your Step** ___
>
> To help your running shoes dry quicker, stuff them with newspaper at the end of the run. You'll be surprised at how this helps soak up the moisture.

Wearing the Right Attire

Layers, layers, and more layers are the secret to staying warm as you train. Frostbite is very real for runners, and you should always cover up well. Wear a hat, and choose something that provides protection for your ears as well. They tend to be very susceptible to the cold. Gloves are another important choice.

Choose your attire to suit your climate; wear several layers and remember that the wicking value of the fabric is an important aspect in keeping you warm. Wicking fabric is made of elements that pull moisture away from the body and help keep it dry. If there is moisture in the air or wind, adjust your outer layer to protect you from that as well. Don't forget to protect your eyes, too; they can get damaged by the winter sun.

If winter running means some snow or rain, then you will need to adjust your shoes. Pick some that have a little more tread, sometimes referred to as road or

> **Road Blocks** ___
>
> Do not put your running shoes next to a heat source (fireplace, radiator, dryer); it will damage the foam your shoes are made of.

trail shoes. Socks for winter running can be thicker than the traditional training pair; be sure to wear them when trying on shoes for winter training. I sometimes suggest increasing your shoe by a half size when you live in a cold climate and wearing thicker socks on a regular basis. And if you do live where you're likely to be getting your feet wet, then you really need a couple pairs of shoes to alternate.

Get Outside and Go

Now that you are dressed properly and ready to go, remember that winter weather will have some real effects on how you train. Staying healthy and injury-free requires that you warm up well, especially in the cold. It's okay to start your warm-up inside, but as you move your run to the great outdoors, be sure to start slowly and adjust as your workout progresses. You won't be able to go as fast or as furious if the weather is bad.

Once you get into your run, you will feel the warmth begin to flow as your body temperature increases. Because of these temperature changes, running on even the coldest day can feel good. I often suggest that runners adjust their routes in the winter to do loops closer to home or the gym, so they can get inside quickly if they need to. Look for paths that are clear of snow and ice, watch your step, take your time, and enjoy the great outdoors.

> **Runner Facts**
>
> Runners sometimes look like the abominable snowman when they run in the winter. When you breathe mostly through your mouth, your breath can freeze on your nose, lips, and/or moustache.

If conditions outside are more than you can tolerate, look for some different workouts in Chapter 8.

Feeling Hot, Hot, Hot: Heat-Related Safety

Let's venture to the other weather extreme that runners face—the heat. If your climate gets hot, then you will need to adjust not only your training patterns to stay injury-free, but also increase your water intake to stay hydrated.

Running in high temperatures can be dangerous. You need to listen to your body and make any necessary adjustments to prevent heat stoke, which can be fatal if it goes too far.

The good news is that the heat usually comes on gradually. It's warm, then warmer, then hot as your training schedules progress. This is good, because it can take your body up to two weeks to become acclimated to training in the heat. So if you are from a milder climate and travel to a hot one, you will need to make even more adjustments.

If you move into a warm climate or start your training during the hot part of the year, build up slowly. I suggest running 1 to 2 miles per day for the first couple of days, then gradually building to 5 to 6 miles during this acclimation period.

The Right Clothes

Summer or heat training requires dressing lightly and wearing light-colored clothes. Pick fabrics that wick away moisture as you sweat and don't absorb it. Your favorite T-shirt doesn't do you any good if it's made from cotton. It will just absorb the moisture, become heavy, and feel yucky as you perspire. I suggest shirts made from 100 percent poly blends; they will keep you cool and dry.

A hat or visor will keep the sun off your head and out of your face. Some runners wear sweat bands to absorb the sweat from around their face, or wrist bands to wipe away sweat as needed. Wear good sunglasses to protect your eyes and cut down on the glare.

The right socks are just as important as the right shoes, and summer running demands ones that don't absorb moisture. Wearing the wrong socks can cause blisters in as little as one training run, and this can set you back on your goals and make even walking painful. Dry your feet right away after a run, and use a foot talc to help absorb moisture.

As at all times of the year, wear the right shoes. Alternate your shoes if you sweat a lot; some models have more breathable fabric than others. Pick a light color, because the dark ones absorb sun and make your feet feel hotter, too.

And remember to protect your skin from the sun! Always put on a good sunscreen before you head out on a daytime run that will last more than 20 minutes. Look for a brand with some waterproof properties that won't come off when you sweat.

Watch Your Step

Avoid salt, alcohol, sweetened drinks, and caffeine during the hot time of the year. These are all diuretics and have a negative effect on your hydration goals.

Also be careful of the type of sunscreen you place on your face. I suggest one of the stick types made for faces (sometimes for children). Too many times I have seen runners reach up to wipe sweat and instead get sunscreen in their eyes. It will bring your run to a screeching halt, and the more your rub, the worse it gets.

If You Don't Beat the Heat, It Will Beat You

I have saved the most important information about running in the heat until last. Hydration is critical. As you run, your core body temperature increases. About 25 percent of the energy you produce during a run is efficient (or being used as part of your metabolism); the other 75 percent is producing heat. This can really put you at risk of heat-related conditions if not carefully managed.

Drink water. Drink lots of water, and not just when you run. Stay hydrated throughout the day. I think everyone has heard that we should have eight full glasses (at least 8 ounces each) every day. It's the minimum you should drink during the course of a day, and if you're training hard, you need even more.

If you are running more than 45 minutes, you should drink some water every 15 to 20 minutes (or one water break during the run and a drink of water before and after the run).

Runs that are shorter than this don't require a water break, but be sure to hydrate before and after the run. Being hydrated aids you in good-quality performances.

Runner Facts

Your urine should be as clear as possible. If your urine is bright yellow, then you are dehydrated—drink more water.

Drink water *while* you run as well. This might seem hard to do, but build a route that will give you some options. Think of stores, restaurants, or public facilities with a water fountain, or spots where you can leave a water bottle that you can access for a drink. The outdoor water hoses from the neighbors can be good choices.

You can always carry water along the way, too: a small water bottle in your hands or a belt that holds a bottle or two. Or if you're seriously training, there are camel backs that lay close on your back and provide needed hydration.

Sports drinks can provide great replenishment for electrolytes; some also contain added protein. These can be helpful in jump-starting you back to hydration, but pay close attention to their calorie content. Often we overlook how many calories these drinks have, and water will usually meet our needs with no added calories.

Watch Your Step

Check the heat index before you head out. It's an indicator of how the temperature and humidity together will impact your run.

Don't ignore the warning signs of heat-related injury or illness while you are running. The three stages of heat illness are cramps, exhaustion, and (the most serious of all) heat stroke. See Chapter 14 for specifics and ways to address it.

Running in hot weather has its own set of challenges. If you manage and plan for it, you can keep your training moving ahead and steer clear of heat-related illness or injury.

Dealing with Inclement Weather

One of my favorite runs is to head out on a fall day where the temperature is about 70 degrees with a light rain falling. The rain drops on my head are refreshing and do nothing except cool me off on this warm day. Too bad that only happens once a year around Colorado.

Rain can pose an added challenge when you head out to run. It creates slippery streets and sidewalks and can make your favorite dirt path a muddy mess. Be sure to wear the correct shoes and adjust your running clothes for the occasion.

Running in a warm-weather rain can be exhausting and a little frustrating, but hardly ever very harmful. Watch for puddles, avoid those you can, and shorten your stride to take fewer and more cautious steps. Try to avoid running in storms that involve lightning. To gauge how far away the lightning is, count after each flash—one one-thousand, two one-thousand—until you hear the thunder. To figure out how far away the lightning is, divide by five; if you count to 20 between the lightning and thunder, then the lightning strike was 4 miles from you.

If you get caught outside as lightning nears, huddle down as close as you can to the ground and stay out from beneath the trees and away from metal objects. And get inside as soon as you can!

The most severe conditions rain can cause come when it's joined by cold temperatures. Hypothermia risks increase when your clothes are wet and the wind is blowing. Layer your running clothes with an outer layer that's some type of waterproof jacket and pants. I have seen runners put plastic bags inside their shoes to give them one more layer of protection from the cold water as well. Choose a hat or cap that will shelter your head and face.

How can you tell if you are getting hypothermia? Shivers are your first sign. If you start to shiver during your run, it's time to turn around and head for a warm shower.

Blown Away

Running in the wind can be a challenge to even the most veteran athlete. There is nothing like a cold headwind to make you want to head right back inside. But if you approach it the right way, you can use the wind during your workout and find a true sense of beating Mother Nature at her own game.

There are two different ways to think of this. If you're the hard-headed, determined type, go right into the wind to start your workout and face the worst first. When you head into the wind first, turning around and having the wind at your back will give you a boost as you complete your workout. Often this type of workout will allow you to have a negative split.

The other approach to wind is to get a ride or drive out and run in one direction with the wind at your back. I often take a van of runners out on the road for whatever distance they are running that day. I drop them off and let them use the wind to push them back into town. This is generally the preferred way to incorporate wind into your workout. It also helps keep the dust and dirt out of your mouth and eyes.

Watch Your Step

Be sure to put some type of lubricant on your cheeks; they can get windburn very quickly. Wear some type of scarf or bandana to cover as much of your face as you can if dust and dirt are blowing strong.

Depending on the temperature, adjust your layers until you get the right combination of coverage. If the wind has a slight chill or is cold, I suggest an outer layer designed to keep the cold wind out and your body heat in.

The Least You Need to Know

◆ Tracks are best for training intervals, not long runs.

◆ If you have access to a trail with wood chips, it's perfect.

◆ Grass is soft to run on, but watch for holes and sprinkler heads.

◆ Cold weather is good to run in, if you stay warm.

◆ If you have to run in high heat, stay hydrated.

Chapter 13

Danger on the Run

In This Chapter

- ◆ Why running on roads is more hazardous than ever
- ◆ Things to take with you on long runs
- ◆ Beware the night
- ◆ Why it is important to beware of local wildlife

When I was a runner going to college in a small town in Arkansas, I would travel to my wife's home community (not large enough to be called a town) and run. There were so many great things that I enjoyed. The roads were generally not crowded, and traffic was considerably slower than the open highway, where large truck and fast cars whiz by you. But even in this environment, I was a foreigner to the locals. Several times during long runs, relatives or nice neighbors would stop and try to give me a ride. Of course, they were just trying to be helpful—why would this city boy be out running country roads if he could get a ride?

This is a great example of how people don't always understand runners. They just don't get why or how we do this. But they're usually the least of our problems! This chapter is about how to run "defensively"—because there are some things you just can't control—and stay safe.

Road-Rage Running

While the kind neighbors living in rural Arkansas were just trying to help out, not every driver feels the same way. There are drivers out there who view the road as their battlefield and will do some fairly outlandish maneuvers to prove their point.

To give you the best odds on dealing with aggressive drivers, always run facing traffic. It gives you the best view of what is happening around you and the widest visual perspective of the traffic risks. Bikers are required to ride with traffic, but runners have a different set of road rules to follow.

> **Watch Your Step**
>
> Listen for cars and get out of their way. Nothing adds insult to injury faster than having a car throw dirty muck all over you as you run in the rain.

Select roads that have wide shoulders and use them. Get over as far as you can and stay out of the path of vehicles. Watch the curves. As vehicles round curves, they often sway over to the side of the road, and if you are too close to highway, it can create a close encounter of the worst kind.

Understand that drivers are sometimes distracted. They are on cell phones, tuning the radio, or maybe just thinking about the million errands they are trying to accomplish. You must stay alert and watch for any signs of distracted driving so you can get out of the way. Pay special attention to weather conditions; even on a clear, bright day, this can be a factor. The afternoon sun beating through a windshield can prevent even a good driver from spotting a runner headed down the road.

Intersections and crosswalks are tools in navigating the roads correctly. But often drivers don't honor the rules as they approach them. Never assume that a car is going to stop or that they will yield to you in the crosswalk. When you're in a battle with someone's car, it won't matter if you're right—you will lose.

During a training run about five years ago, a group of my male athletes were pelted by water balloons and bottles that a rowdy group of kids decided to throw as they crossed paths with the athletes. The athletes were immediately angered and wanted to chase down the car and retaliate. Thank goodness they came to their senses before something even more serious ensued. You never know who might be in the car or what they might be capable of doing.

 Road Blocks

If you run in a group:

♦ Don't run next to each other. Single file is the safest way as you head down the road.

♦ Don't just blindly follow each other. Everyone should stay alert and always yield to vehicles.

♦ Don't give in to peer pressure and do something that doesn't work for you.

♦ If you hear threats or jeers, keep moving and ignore them.

We would all like to think that we could live in harmony with our fellow community members and that no one would take offense at our need to work up a sweat or lose a few pounds, but those misguided drivers do exist.

When you encounter an aggressive driver, get out of his or her way. Don't make any gestures or shout anything—it will only inflame the driver and worsen the confrontation. If an aggressive driver swerves at you or threatens you, call the police and report the person. We have a duty to get these types of drivers off the roads.

The Night Doesn't Belong to Runners

I believe that running is a daylight event. So many things can go wrong at night that your risk of injury increases substantially.

However, if you find yourself with no other choice, then take all the precautions you can. Wear reflective clothing, choose lighted paths, and run loops that are close to homes or businesses that you know well.

In Their Shoes

College running programs have rules established by their governing bodies (Adams State's is the NCAA) that set boundaries and rules for all of our athletic programs and provide protections and guaranteed rest and time off for the athletes. One of these rules is what most coaches and athletes refer to as the "NCAA day off"—the day where coaches are not allowed to meet and work with their athletes. Most athletes run on their own at a time that best suits them, using this day as their opportunity to catch up with school work, socializing, and so on.

A dear friend of mine coaches in the Los Angeles area (Irvine, to be exact) at a small private college. It is located in a safe, rather affluent neighborhood, and going out for a run seems like a pretty low risk. A few years ago, on his team's NCAA day, one of his athletes set out for a run on her own. As she headed off campus and down through the town, she began unwinding, focusing on the thoughts in her head versus paying attention to the environment around her. As she neared where she wanted to cross the street, she took a quick glance back and stepped out into the road.

That's the moment the car hit her. She didn't even see it coming. As she lay unconscious in a local hospital for well over four hours, no one knew who she was. She hadn't brought any identification with her, thus leaving the authorities with a difficult puzzle. She was several miles away from school when she was hit, and nobody could identify her. Thankfully, she regained consciousness later that day and was able to give her name and how to contact persons who could assist and support her.

After learning of this experience, I tell my runners that they should always carry some form of ID with them. Even the old tip of putting your name and address on the inside of your shoe will help. Think ahead and plan for the unexpected.

Two's Company

Running is one of those great activities that you can enjoy alone or with company. I suggest doing as many runs as you can with a group or at least one other runner. When you share the road with someone, you improve your chances of finishing the workout safe and sound. Partner running can protect you both from personal danger or from something as simple as a fall that leaves you unable to hobble home.

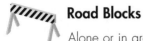

Road Blocks _____

> Alone or in groups, I strongly suggest following some basic safety
> rules to improve your chances of staying injury- or accident-free:
>
> ◆ Run in an area where you can be seen and heard if some-
>   thing happens.
> ◆ Consider a loop route that takes you close to home several
>   times.
> ◆ Let someone know you are heading out on a run; tell them
>   how long you plan to be gone and the route you are taking.
> ◆ Consider carrying a cell phone.
> ◆ Consider a whistle.
> ◆ Stay away from trails that are hidden by brush or trees.
> ◆ Alter your route, and don't become too predictable.

Headset and mp3 players are a reality in our running world. I read
all the time how runners shouldn't wear them, but I see runners with
them every day. The reasons to leave them home are very compelling.
Having earphones on greatly inhibits your ability to hear the world
around you, and you may not hear any warning signs before you cross
into the wrong path. If you insist on wearing them anyway, use good
judgment. Wear them only when running on trails or tracks, where
you'll be less likely to cross paths with a car.

Another item to leave home is jewelry. It doesn't serve any purpose in
running and can give a would-be robber a motive that you don't want.
Besides, I've seen runners lose valuable jewelry during a run, and the
chances for recovery are extremely slim.

I'm sometimes asked if I suggest running with mace. I really don't.
From what I've heard, mace usually ends up being used on runners and
pedestrians, not by them, and does more harm than good.

When Animals Attack

While runners are often dog lovers, you won't find many runners who
love being chased by a dog. If you find yourself on the wrong side of
an aggressive dog, slow down, walk, or consider coming to a complete

stop. A dog's instinct is to chase and attack. If you take the chase element out of the equation, it may be all that is necessary to send Fido heading home.

Don't make eye contact or any other threatening gestures. Dogs interpret these as aggressive and will respond accordingly. Keep the dog within your sights, but try walking away. Be boring; if you don't react, then maybe the dog will lose interest.

If all this fails and you are attacked, then hit the ground, roll up into a ball and cover your throat and face with your arms and hands. Dogs will try to go for soft tissue areas and your neck and face are very vulnerable.

Yell as loud as possible, get someone's attention, and have them assist you. Once the attack has ended, seek medical attention. It's important to have your rabies shots up to date or to get one right away if you need it. Identify the dog and contact the owner to see if the dog is current on his shots as well. Rabies is still a risk when bitten by a dog. Report any dog incidents to law enforcement and protect yourself and others from any future attacks.

Bear Country Safari

Finding yourself face to face with a bear while on a run can be frightening. Bears rarely exhibit aggressive behavior, and it is even rarer for them to attack. But anything can happen, and knowing the right way to handle it can certainly change the outcome. Most likely your encounter with a bear will be a short but thrilling view of the animal.

If you're running in bear country, make some noise along the way. Generally a bear will hear you and stay off your path. This is the kind of run where you want a partner along to talk with; it's both social and safer. Being quiet as you glide through the woods may bring you face to face with a startled bear. If you do see a bear, respect its need for space and stay back. Make a detour to another route and clear the area.

Always remain calm and access the situation. Bears will react more defensively if startled or they are protecting cubs. Make sure the bear knows you are a human by talking in a normal tone, outstretching your arms and waving them around to make yourself appear larger. Try to move upwind to get out of the bear's line of smell.

The bear may swat the ground or make a short jab toward you. Don't panic; these are usually just bear gestures to let you know it doesn't want any company. If you are attacked, fight back with all your might. Putting up as much fight as possible will encourage the bear to give up and back off. Use sticks, rocks, or whatever else you can put your hands on as a weapon toward the bear.

These tips are for encounters with a black bear, the most common bears found in the United States. If you have the unfortunate experience of running into a grizzly bear, then you should not fight back, but instead "play dead" so that the grizzly bear will lose interest.

Mountain Lions

Those of us who live in the western United States are thrilled when we get a rare glimpse of a mountain lion (also known as a cougar, panther, or puma). But if you encounter one during a run, the thrill can turn to fear very quickly. As with bears, try to run through mountain lion country with a partner. Making any noise will generally keep the mountain lion far from your path.

If you do come face to face with a big cat, do not approach them. They will view any attempts to come near them or their young as a threat. Keep your eye on the animal, and try to appear as large as possible. Wave your arms and throw rocks or sticks to intimidate the mountain lion and reduce your attractiveness as a target. Be extra careful that you don't turn your back or bend down in the view of the mountain lion. That is interpreted as a sign of weakness and could provoke an attack.

Be sure to report any sightings to the proper officials, thus allowing them to give fair warning to other runners.

Coyotes

I would rank coyotes as a fairly low threat to runners, as they tend to be much more afraid of us than we are of them. But recently in Denver, a coyote attacked a group of children playing near a running path and hurt one young girl pretty badly. I think as the coyote's food sources are depleted and we move more into their domain, the threat of attacks may increase.

Know that the coyote is most active around dawn or dusk; they are usually scavenging for food. Like other wild animals, they will retreat when faced with a large, aggressive person. Wave your arms; throw rocks or sticks; and, if you are attacked, fight back aggressively.

Snakes

As you wind along your running path, coming face to face with a rattlesnake will make your heart skip a beat. You should stop, assess your situation, and adjust your path well around the snake. I have known runners who just keep right on going, even thinking of jumping right over the snake (or actually doing it). Any harassment or attempts to move the snake will set off its aggressive nature and you could find yourself with a snakebite. Snakes can move quickly and strike much further away from the ground than you think.

If you are unlucky enough to get bitten, seek medical help right away. Antidotes are the only real treatment for snake bites, and you need professional assistance with these treatments.

Remember, when you run, you're entering the habitat of many creatures. Staying aware and understanding their behavior patterns will go a long way in keeping you safe and injury-free.

The Least You Need to Know

◆ Never take on a car, or its driver.

◆ If you're running, learn about the animals in that area you might encounter on a run.

◆ No matter what happens, keep your composure.

Part 4

Listen When Your Body Talks

Do you know what leads to most injuries? Not knowing what causes them, and thus not being prepared. But sometimes injuries are just inevitable. In this final part, we'll talk about what they are and which ones are serious, in a gathering of maladies to watch for from head to toe. We'll get real and address the difference between soreness and pain, and when pain means injury. Most little nagging things can be smartly managed. Like everything else in life, prevention is the best cure!

I'll share some ideas for cross-training when you need a break or want to keep up your cardiovascular fitness while you work through an injury or illness. Finally if you're an overachiever—and you probably are if you picked up this book to make your life better—then we need to talk about how motivation and inspiration, properly utilized, can help you reach your highest goals.

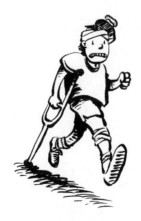

Chapter 14

The Book on Running Injuries

In This Chapter

- ◆ What to do when the obstacle is physical
- ◆ How to cope with common ailments
- ◆ Spotting lifelong issues you can minimize
- ◆ How to best put back issues behind you

Every runner has experienced a few of the injuries or ailments that come along with this sport. Often these are minor, such as blisters or chafing, but they can occasionally turn ugly and become an injury that holds you back from your running or reaching your racing goals.

We rarely sustain running injuries from just one factor; most often a combination of things bring them on. There usually isn't a quick fix for an injury, either, as many injuries come from what we call chronic overuse. However, there are ways to prevent them, and the best way is with your brain. Develop your understanding of what your body is telling you, and you'll know what you're up against.

I have tried to list some of the most common injuries and give you a little background info and suggestions on how to take care of them. The best advice I can give you is to use common sense when it comes to injuries. Training while you are hurt will only make matters worse and, in some extreme cases, might have a disastrous effect over the long haul. If you don't see improvements within a reasonable time, seek medical attention. It's better to be safe than sorry.

When Pain Stops Gains

One of the most misused phrases in the history of training and sports is "no pain, no gain." It's important to differentiate pain from exhaustion or physical stress and pain that is because of a broken bone, torn muscle, or a serious physiological issue that can actually kill someone (dehydration on a hot day, or heat exhaustion). As you train and get to know your body better, you'll know what real pain should and should not feel like, and how to take precautions.

Pain usually means that gains aren't in your immediate future, so find out what's going on before you decide to "push through it," because if it's something serious, you'll only make it worse. You certainly don't want to hear this line: "It's going to take time—along with therapy and rehab—to get you back out on that road." You've gone all these miles, put in all kinds of time, made a lot of progress, and you believe that if you have to slow down, your progress is going to stop. But it doesn't have to be that way.

Once you're able to recognize the common running injuries, then a methodical approach and self-treatment plan can keep you from worsening your injury and sometimes help you avoid injury altogether.

It's important to catch these injuries early. Usually you let warning signs go unaddressed, like little pains that subside after your run or don't seem serious enough to ice or take a day off. When you catch these injuries and treat them early, you can effectively manage them and get back to running ASAP.

Overuse Injuries

If you sustain an overuse injury, you probably increased your distance or speed too soon, or were training too many hard days in a row. These are commonly called training errors. The repetitive motion involved in the sport will cause 70 percent of runners to develop an overuse injury this year. You need to learn the warning signs and precautions to take to ward them off. If you have already sustained an overuse injury, then I will share the most effective measures for dealing with it.

Acute Injuries

If you're out running and step in a hole or on a rock, you will join the multitudes who have sustained an acute strain or sprain of muscle tissue. It is very important to allow this type of injury adequate time to heal before resuming your training; an acute injury can very quickly turn into a chronic one. If your injury isn't too severe and you treat it properly, it can be corrected in a matter of days. If it's severe and goes untreated, it can take months to heal properly. These injuries are also common, but you can prevent some of them with better stretching and muscle strengthening. Sometimes, however, it's just plain bad luck.

Anemia

If you have anemia, your blood isn't carrying enough oxygen to your muscles, brain, or any part of the rest of your body. Anemia in runners is most commonly caused by not having enough iron in your blood. Your blood needs iron to make hemoglobin, an iron-rich protein. It also carries oxygen from your lungs to the rest of your body.

Your iron could be low as a result of several factors, any one or a combination of which can increase your risk of anemia. These include heavy periods, pregnancy, ulcers, colon problems, or a diet lacking in iron, such as vegetarians often have. You can also get anemia from not getting enough folic acid or vitamin B_{12}.

Anemia symptoms include feeling out of breath on routine hard workouts, or feeling weak, cold, dizzy, or irritable. Anemia is usually confirmed with a blood test; be sure the doctor knows you're a runner. Ask to have your ferritin level tested, as this is the best indication for runners. Ferritin is a test that providers order to see how much iron your body has stored for future use. The test is done, usually with an iron test and the TIBC, to learn about iron levels in your blood. Ferritin is the best test for iron deficiency and a very good test for iron overload. Treatment depends on the kind of anemia you have.

Exercise-Induced Asthma

If you experience coughing, wheezing, chest tightness, or chest pain only minutes after you begin running, you may have exercise-induced asthma (EIA). EIA affects different runners in varying degrees. Asthma affects roughly 7 percent of the American population, and the majority of these have additional problems with strenuous exercise.

If you have EIA, then you've noticed by now that you're very sensitive to temperature and humidity changes. If you breathe through your mouth instead of a combination of mouth and nose, this won't allow for any warming of the air before it passes through your lower bronchial passages. Breathing through your nose will humidify the air to 80 to 90 percent relative humidity; mouth breathing will only humidify the air to 60 to 70 percent. If the air is colder and drier, it tends to increase hacking and wheezing symptoms.

Have a doctor test you. This will usually include a breathing test while resting, a field breathing test, and a look at your history with breathing problems. If you experience breathing difficulties after only a few minutes, or your airflow is reduced 10 to 20 percent postexercise, then you may be considered positive for EIA.

Treatment will often include taking medication through inhalers. These medications (albuterol, pirbuterol, or terbutaline) have proven very useful for 75 to 90 percent of patients who have EIA. Effects of these medicines usually last for four to six hours. I personally have coached numerous All-Americans and even national champions who have EIA. If you're treated properly, you can still excel; if you go untreated, you can really struggle.

The Sprain of Pain: Ankles

You don't even have to run to get an ankle sprains, but if you do run, you need to learn the best way to take care of it. Ankle sprains can happen just as easy as stepping on a twig. Basically a sprain is the over-stretching of ligaments in the ankle. In some severe cases there is tearing of the ligament tissue.

Typically these sprains happen when we are running on trail or uneven path, but they can happen just as easily on a smooth surface. Most often the sprain occurs as the toe is on the ground and the heel is in an up position; this creates tension or torque on the ligaments in the ankle.

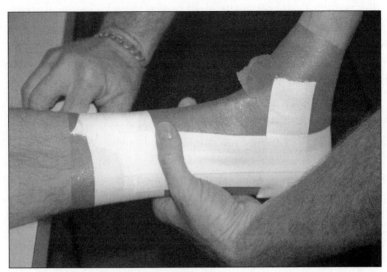

Sprained ankles require constant maintenance.

Once you sprain your ankle, it is important that you stop running and apply ice immediately. Trying to finish your workout can make matters much worse. The swelling will depend largely on how severely you sprained it, but if you can apply ice immediately, you can reduce the bleeding and swelling that occurs and reduce the time it will take to heal. You should also elevate the injury, which will also limit bleeding and swelling.

Depending on the level of sprain, it could take a day or two or several weeks for the pain and swelling to subside. After this period, you can begin therapy and strengthening exercises. Be sure to complete all rehab and strengthening work, as the ankle will be more susceptible to sprains if you don't finish your rehab work.

Achilles Tendonitis

This is another one of those "if you run long enough, you're sure to get it" injuries. Tendonitis is one of the most frequent running-related injuries; it can affect almost any area of the body, but is most commonly found in the Achilles, knee, and foot. Tendonitis is a classic overuse injury; as you begin to pile on those miles, add speed work, or do more hill work, you increase your risk of tendonitis.

Achilles tendonitis is one of the most severe types. It's typically caused by overworking or overstretching the Achilles. The Achilles is more prone to injury when you increase running volume or intensity. Hill running, long runs, and speed work are definite no-nos if you're having Achilles problems.

Watch Your Step

Try this simple trick for dealing with an overstretched Achilles: put a heel lift in your shoe (usually some piece of firm rubber works great); this will lesson the stretch on the already overstretched Achilles. Many times I will see younger and/or beginning runners wear shoes without enough support or cushion in the heel. This can lead to Achilles problems as well.

You can usually find good heel lifts at your local pharmacy or grocery stores. If you are looking for a higher end selection, then look to a sports goods store. Depending on the severity of your injury, you may want to have a heel lift custom made. Comfort can usually be achieved by adding between a $\frac{1}{8}$- to $\frac{3}{8}$-inch heel lift.

The Achilles tendon actually slides through a tube and hooks the two muscles of the calf to the bottom of your heel. Despite all the work you do with strengthening your calves, the tube that the Achilles passes through remains the same size. If your Achilles tendon becomes swollen and the tube stays the same size, this will usually cause additional friction and pain. You must be very careful with this injury as you can end up with a torn or ruptured Achilles.

The worst thing you can do with any significant Achilles pain is continue running. Even running on grass and soft surfaces can make matters worse. You still want to avoid hard surfaces such as concrete because those are just bad for you in general, but overly soft grass isn't good for those with Achilles pain, either. Therefore, you will want to find a firm level surface; something like a dirt road without rocks or gravel would work just fine.

Arthritis and Running

As a coach for more than 20 years, I am frequently asked if running can cause arthritis. You would think that all the pounding of the pavement, training session after training session, race after race, would cause wear and tear on your hips, knees, and joints.

The truth of the matter is that running does not cause arthritis. But before you get too excited, you must also know that if you already have arthritis, then running can certainly make your arthritis condition worse.

Running creates significant stress on the body, especially the knees, hips, and ankles. The total impact with each stride can be four to six times your body weight; if you have arthritis this can be very harmful, hastening the wear and tear to your knees and joints. This problem can be further exacerbated if you are overweight and running on pavement or concrete.

If you have arthritis and decide that running is still for you, then you should find as soft a surface to run on as possible, and consult your physician on any medications you may need to take. You should also avoid downhill running and speed work. But remember, running does *not* cause arthritis if your knees are healthy and normal.

Back Pain

Lower back pain is usually caused by two or three different problems. Your abdominal or back muscles could be too weak, creating an imbalance that causes pulling and shifting in your lower back. You may have overly tight hamstrings, which will cause more pulling to occur, this time on the hips, which can cause the lower back to shift out of place. Finally, having an imbalance of the feet or leg length can also cause unnatural stride patterns and shifting of weight from one leg to the other.

The bottom line is that they all are a big pain in the butt! I mean back! If your back pain does not feel worse after you run, it's probably OK to continue. But you may want to cut back on the miles you put in. You may also want to stay away from hill runs, as this can exacerbate the problems. As you run up and down hills, changes occur in your posture that put a greater strain on your back.

As a coach, before I even begin trying to address someone's back problem, I will ask, "How did you hurt your back?" Sometimes this gives me a better idea of how to correct the problem. Sometimes your back can begin hurting after wearing a brand-new pair of shoes, or maybe your shoes are way too old. It could be that big box that you moved for your boss.

If you just hurt your back, ice should be your first treatment. The ice will bring some relief to an acute injury of the back, in case you need to stop any bleeding that can happen with small muscle tears or strains. If the problem is more chronic, apply heat first, massage, then ice. If this does not bring relief, you may look into having your doctor prescribe low frequency e-stim from a physical therapist. E-stim or electrical stimulation is most commonly used to control pain. The stimulation helps reduce the tightness in the injury. It also can improve the recovery time for an injury.

Regardless, some of the better methods in dealing with back pain include using damp or moist heat, including heat packs, hot baths, hot showers, and steam rooms. Oftentimes massaging the lower back, starting at the base of the lower back and working upward, can bring significant relief.

One area that is often overlooked in lower back pain is strengthening of the abdominal and back muscles. These spinal erectors protect the spinal column and hold it in place. We use a lot of exercises to strengthen the lower back, including hyperextensions and an exercise as simple as lying flat on the floor on the stomach and raising the right arm and left leg at the same time, switching, and repeating.

Another good exercise is lying flat on your back with your knees raised, then pushing your lower back to touch the ground and holding for a 10- to 15-second count, repeating three times. The final exercise is called the parachute; it looks just like it sounds. While lying face down, simultaneously lift your arms and chest, and upper and lower legs off the ground. Hold this for 10 to 15 seconds, and repeat three times.

Sometimes you can alleviate your back pain with an adjustment from a chiropractor. Sometimes you just need a different pair of shoes. And sometimes it just takes plain old time to heal the core, or center, of our bodies. I hope that one of these remedies will work for you.

Sciatica

If you feel pain in your lower back and it runs down through your butt into the backs of your leg, you probably have sciatic nerve problems. The sciatic nerve is a horsetail-shaped nerve that comes out of the lower lumbar region and splits at the buttocks area and continues down both legs, ending at the feet.

If your sciatic nerve hurts, it's usually being pinched in the lower lumbar region, where it splits around the tailbone. This pain can continue to worsen as the disks in the lower lumbar region become compacted. Your spine shortens or becomes more compact as you go through your daily routine, and any activity that involves pounding (like running) increases this compacting. As your vertebrae become compacted, it increases the likelihood of the sciatic nerve being pinched.

Sometimes you can feel the nerve pain at specific locations in your leg or butt. This pain usually begins as mild discomfort but can often get much worse if left untreated. This pain will often begin or become worse after a hard workout or hill session; it can become particularly bad after long runs.

Watch Your Step

Suggestions for dealing with sciatic nerve pain:

- If you have severe sciatic pain, do not run or use the stair-climbing machine for a least a week.
- Take nonsteroidal anti-inflammatory drugs (NSAIDS) for one week.
- Ice your lower back for 15 minutes, at least five to six times a day.
- Strengthen your abdominal and buttock muscles.

To deal with this problem we try to stretch out the lower back area with a lot of sit-and-reach stretches. We also do some inversion stretching with hanging devices. Another excellent treatment is acupressure on the bottom of the foot, specifically the heel area, working from the middle to the outside, where the sciatic nerve actually ends. Massaging this area of your foot stimulates the nerve and can rejuvenate it.

You can alleviate some of your problems by changing your sleeping habits. Sleeping on your stomach will irritate your sciatica. You should also sleep on a firm mattress. If you sleep on your back, put a pillow underneath your knees. If you sleep on your side, then place a pillow between your knees.

Neck Pain

Muscle tightness is the main cause of neck injuries. Neck tightness can create so much pain that you can't walk comfortably, much less run. The solution is restoring normal range of motion and restoring the regular curvature and position of the spine. In mild cases, this will require stretching, heat, and time off. In more severe cases, therapy could be added to the treatment.

If you have an acute injury to the neck, ice can be very beneficial. Runners are more susceptible to neck problems because of the impact and compression of the spine with each stride. This process increases the possibility of neck pain and muscle tightness. Therefore, if you have a good chiropractor, visit him or her often to keep those neck blues away.

Hip Flexor Pain

If you have pain in your hip, it's most likely caused by overuse of the muscles that allow you to lift your knee and bend at the waist. Overusing these tendons can cause them to be inflamed and cause tendonitis. Your symptoms will usually include pain in the groin and pain where your thigh meets your pelvis.

You can prevent a hip flexor strain by warming up properly and doing specific stretching exercises before your run. If you're going out for a hard run, don't rush or skip through the warm-up and stretching, as this is your best prevention.

If you have hip flexor pain, your best options are icing, taking an anti-inflammatory, and rehab exercises. If treated properly with rest, often you can return to running in two to three days. Be patient; this injury can be very frustrating, but if your push through it, it may cause you to have to take additional time off.

If you're recovering from a hip flexor injury, switch to a low-impact activity that doesn't make your hip feel worse. Try swimming instead of running for a few days.

Side Stitch

Almost all of us get these pesky side stitches at one time or another. Sometimes they're mild, but sometimes they can bring your run to a crawl. Only recently have scientists been able to explain the cause of these annoying side stitches: overstretching of ligaments in the abdomen caused by the pounding of running while breathing in and out.

 Watch Your Step

Dealing with a side stitch:
1. Stretching the area in pain can help alleviate the side stitch.
2. Slow down and jog until the pain lessens or subsides.
3. Drink water to hydrate before you run.
4. Massage and/or press on the area you feel pain.

Runners typically breathe every two to four steps. Most runners breathe out as their left foot touches the ground, but some breathe out as their right foot touches the ground. If you breathe out as your right foot touches the ground, this can cause greater impact on the liver (on the right).

It is believed that this repeated stretching of the ligament that holds the liver in place can cause spasms (side stitches) to occur. Stop running and place your hand on the right side of your abdomen and push up. This will lift the liver slightly; continue to breathe normally, and hopefully your pain will diminish.

Agony of "De Feet"

Your feet are your wheels, and like tires on a car, they're often the first things to feel the impact of the road. Here are some common foot ailments and treatments.

Black Toenail

One of the first injuries you may have—especially if you are just beginning or getting back into running—is "black toenail." What usually happens is that your shoes are too small or too large and your foot moves inside your shoe, which creates added pressure and or banging on the toe, causing bleeding under the toenail. The toe begins to protect itself and fills with fluid under the toenail.

> **Road Blocks**
>
> Shoes are a key for runners, but another important element is the sock. An ill-fitting sock or one made of the wrong material can cause serious issues, some related to hygiene but also from the stress an improper material or size can cause on the toes, heels, and Achilles area.

Black toenails are commonly caused by athletes who step up volume and start to increase running on hard surfaces. Hot weather can also be a factor in black toe. Most commonly it's a combination of stepping up the training and perhaps an issue with tight socks and/or shoes.

Depending on how much pressure and how painful it feels, you might not have to do anything. Your body is protecting itself with the fluid under the nail and you really don't want to risk infection.

However, if the pressure is creating significant pain and you want to continue running, you could seek medical attention and have a small hole drilled in your toenail, which will relieve the blood and fluid—and pressure—from under the toenail. You will feel instantly better. Be sure to watch for any signs of infection.

Hammer Toe and Claw Toe

Next time you try on those high-heeled, fashionable shoes, be careful. Looks can be deceiving. These shoes can be beautiful, but they can also create problems for your feet. Hammer toes and/or claw toes can develop in runners and nonrunners alike, and usually come from a mixture of reasons.

Hammer toe is just what it sounds like: it is when a toe folds up permanently at the middle joint. In general, hammer toe can result from years of wearing shoes that are too small and as a result cause muscle imbalances in your toes. Claw toe is when your toe is bound/cramped up like a clenched fist. Claw toe can also be caused by wearing small shoes, as well as alcoholism and/or diabetes.

How do we know what shoe size is too small? If your shoes don't allow adequate space for your toes and they are being pushed together, then the shoes are too small. This will eventually lead to hammer toe and/or claw toe. Many fashionable shoes made today are too narrow for comfort and don't allow for proper biomechanics of the foot. These shoes are made for looks, not practical use. If at all possible, leave them on the rack and find something that feels as good as it looks.

If your hammer toe is caught early enough, it can be treated without surgery. The usual treatment would include wearing shoes that provide plenty of space for your toes, and completing toe stretches. If you complete these treatments successfully, your toes could return to normal. If you have chronic hammer toe, then surgery may be necessary.

> **Watch Your Step**
>
> If you are one of those runners who suffer with hammer or claw toe, look to a trained professional for guidance in selecting an athlete shoe that fits you properly. If your condition becomes serious, consult a podiatrist.

If you suffer from claw toe, similar stretches are prescribed. In severe cases of claw toe, you will need to find a shoe that has more room in the toe box, or order custom-made shoes to fit your foot appropriately. Sometimes you can add special pads in your shoes to lessen pressure on your toes.

Ingrown Toenail

Almost everyone will have an ingrown toenail sooner or later. This usually happens as a result of cutting your toenail to short or the toe box of your shoes placing too much pressure on your toenails. This causes your toenail to cut and grow into the surrounding skin tissue.

Start the treatment for ingrown toenail by wearing shoes that don't put pressure on the toe and allowing enough room for the toes to not rub.

Also, soaking the toe in warm water and not trimming the toenail at all (or too short) allows the toe to heal.

If these remedies don't bring you relief, then you may need surgical removal of the toenail. It can be done at some doctor's offices with a little anesthesia. Most of the time you will feel immediate relief once the toenail is removed. However, you will need to allow the toe to heal properly before beginning to train again. If the toenail requires extensive work to remove, be sure to follow all the post-treatment directions.

Plantar Fasciitis

The plantar fascia is a long fibrous tissue that runs from the heel to the forefoot. The purpose of this tissue is to provide support for joints, bones, and muscles of the foot during midstep. You can continue to run, but proceed with caution. Begin treatments to alleviate the tightness; if this injury becomes chronic it will start a chain reaction that will eventually affect your running form. (Plantar fascia can turn into a heel spur that may eventually require surgery.

Plantar fascia treatment is no fun.

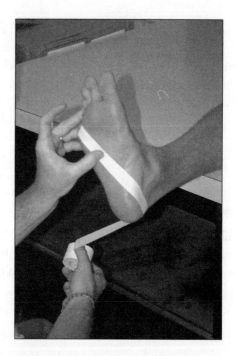

Several factors contribute to plantar fasciitis: increasing mileage and intensity too quickly, increasing hill workouts, wearing spikes, running on sloped surfaces, and running on too hard or too soft surfaces.

I know you've heard this one before: An ounce of prevention is worth a pound of cure. The best way to deal with plantar fasciitis is to never get it in the first place. It is vital to have good shoes that fit your foot. By that I mean shoes made for your arch type, and if you have a high arch, you definitely need the right fit for your foot.

Pay attention to the types of surfaces (asphalt, concrete, grass, dirt) and slants (uphill, downhill, crowned, or sloped) you are running on. Adapt slowly to any new surfaces you add to your training regimen. I suggest no more than 10 percent increases in volume or 5 percent in intensity, as this will help you prevent plantar fasciitis.

But if you've got it, what do you do about it? Your best alternative is to decrease your mileage by 25 to 50 percent, if not take a break from running altogether. If you continue running, try to avoid speed work, wearing shoes with little or no support (spikes)—and if you see a hill, turn the other direction.

Icing the plantar fascia for 5 to 10 minutes can reduce the swelling; it's smart to ice multiple times a day, but don't ice for any longer than 10 minutes at a time. Next time you do, try it this way: Freeze water in a plastic bottle, lay the bottle on the ground, and roll your foot on it from the ball to the heel, going back and forth, and continuing that protocol for 5 to 10 minutes. This treatment will stretch and ice it at the same time. I will have my runners alternate the frozen water bottle with a tennis ball. The tennis ball also increases the flexibility in that tendon. You can then progress to a harder ball, something like a baseball or even a golf ball, but don't start with a hard ball, as your plantar is very tender.

Quite a bit of research has shown that you can limit plantar fascia problems through flexibility and strengthening of the foot and calf. If you get it, treat it quickly and get rid of it. You don't want any injury, but this is one you surely need to avoid.

Athlete's Foot

It sounds like a compliment, but it's not anything you would ever want. Athlete's foot is a skin disease caused by fungus. If you do get it, most times it appears between your toes first. This fungus commonly attacks your feet because your shoes create the ideal environment (warm and damp) for this fungus to thrive. It was appropriately named as it is often contracted in showers, locker rooms, and other athletic facilities.

If you do get this fungus, the symptoms include dry itchy skin, scaling, inflammation, and blisters. Many times the blisters will itch and as you scratch them it causes the blisters to break; this can lead to cracking of the skin, pain, and swelling. It's not very comfortable—and, even worse, it can easily spread to other warm, damp areas (groin and underarms).

Runner Facts

To beat athlete's foot:

- ◆ Use shower shoes when showering in athletic or public locker rooms.
- ◆ Use talcum powder on your feet and in your shoes to keep moisture away.
- ◆ Wear dry socks and change socks frequently if your feet sweat a lot.

In order to treat this fungus effectively, it is best to use a fungicidal chemical that is most commonly sold as a topical cream. It is also important to wash your feet often and completely dry them, between each toe, before putting your dry socks back on.

If you have a hard time getting rid of this fungus or it lasts longer than two weeks, consult your doctor or podiatrist.

Blisters

Blisters are another common issue for runners, especially if you're just starting out. Blistering is one reason why shoe selection is so important, and why breaking in your shoes and wearing appropriate socks are also critical factors. If you aren't wearing a well-fitted shoe, you'll have lots of friction, whether the shoe is too small or too big. Proper socks are also important.

If you do get a blister, the best thing to do is let it heal itself, especially if you don't have to run right away or it's not too uncomfortable. The body, once again, is trying to heal itself, and the liquid underneath the blister is trying to protect it from infections. But if the blister is painful, you may want to release the pressure by boiling a needle for 5 to 10 minutes, then carefully pierce the blister. After popping the blister, press all the fluid out, then use antiseptic cream to prevent infection and cover the area with a bandage.

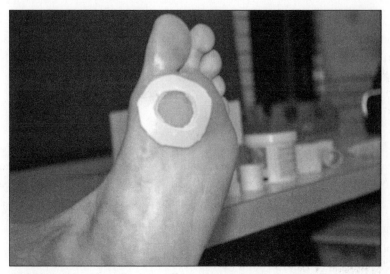

2nd Skin and a "donut" are an effective treatment.

2nd Skin and other like products are a type of bandage that is skinlike in appearance and texture. It helps prevent blisters and other sensitive areas from getting rubbed raw or infected. However, after training, make sure you clean the area and even apply a new piece of 2nd Skin the next time you run.

A donut bandage is typically a round foam pad with a hole in the middle. The hole should be slightly larger than the blister and this will provide cushioning and space for the blister by eliminating the friction when you walk or run.

Calluses

Calluses are another common problem—anyone who runs for any significant amount of time has dealt with calluses to some degree, including yours truly. Calluses usually develop as a result of pressure points on areas of the foot. The shape of your foot and your skin type are big contributing factors.

As a preventive measure, you can put lubricants like petroleum jelly on your feet to reduce friction and avoid calluses. If you do have calluses, don't let them get large. When calluses get too big, you can develop blood blisters underneath, which can magnify your problem.

Try to moisten your feet to soften up the callus. Also use a pumice stone to remove some of the callus to prevent buildup—because once you get buildup it does create other problems. Your podiatrist can trim your calluses as well, but trimming can be tedious and cause soreness, so deal with them before they get to the point they need trimming.

Stone Bruise

If you've had stone bruises on the bottom of your feet, you undoubtedly know they can become very painful. These bruises are generally caused by stepping on hard objects and are just like other bruises you can get.

The difference between a stone bruise on your foot and a bruise on your leg is that you have to keep landing on your foot. Stone bruises are extremely difficult to heal unless you stay off your feet for a couple of days.

If you're in this predicament, swimming is a good alternative workout. This will allow you to get your workout in while staying off that bruise. Biking is okay, but only if you keep the part of your foot with a stone bruise off the pedal. You may consider moving your foot to the middle of your pedal, as stone bruises usually occur at the forefoot or heel area.

Skin Conditions

You'll be surprised how rough running is on your skin—on your face, hands, and all over your body.

Cuts and Scrapes

The line from *Field of Dreams* is, "If you build it, he will come." In running we often say, "If you run, you will fall." If you run long enough, you will fall at least a few times, resulting in cuts, scrapes, and bruises. These can vary significantly depending on the surface you're running on that day.

A nasty fall can leave you with cuts, scrapes, road burn, and a bruised ego. Clean the area with soap, water, and a soft washcloth. Avoid getting the soap in the actual cut, as that will irritate the wound. Clean all around the cuts or scrapes, then rinse with water to cleanse the area of any dirt or debris.

If the cut or scrape is bleeding (bleeding helps clean the wound), apply gentle pressure with a clean gauze or cloth. If your cut continues to bleed and it is on your arms or legs, elevate your arm or leg above your heart to slow the bleeding. If bleeding continues and soaks your bandage, don't remove the bandage as this can increase the bleeding; just add layers on top of one another until it stops bleeding.

Once the wound has been cleaned and there is no bleeding, you can cover it with a bandage or adhesive strip. Some wounds won't need to be covered if there is no risk of irritation or infection. Yet others (large scrapes) may need to be covered and kept moist with a protective bandage. Your doctor can give you the best advice.

Although most small cuts and scrapes will heal fine without antibiotic creams and ointments, these creams can reduce the chance of infection and promote healing; you should use these ointments when appropriate. Once your cut or scrape develops a scab, be sure to leave it on as this is the body's own type of bandage. This scab will continue to keep your wound clean.

I would like to add a word of caution, just common sense when examining a cut. Too often runners take the fall, cover the wound, and wait for it to heal, when what the injury really needed was a thorough cleaning and a few stitches. Be smart: avoiding the stitches can sometimes multiply the recovery time when an infection shows up. If you can see into the wound or the gap in the skin is wide, seek medical attention.

Chafing

Imagine yourself having a great run; you're feeling good and the weather is great. Then you notice an irritation under your arm. Minutes later, it seems like someone took sandpaper and is going to town under your arm. That's how quickly chafing seems to happen. It's definitely irritating, no pun intended.

The main contributing factors of chafing are sweat and friction. As your body tries to cool itself off, you're probably sweating pretty good, leaving sodium crystals and friction to work their wonders. It actually does feel like sandpaper if you continue running after the problem starts.

There are several ways to prevent chafing. You might start with trying to stay extra dry by using powders to absorb your sweat.

Watch Your Step

If you have sensitive nipples, you can place athletic tape or an adhesive bandage over them to avoid chafing there.

Something else about chafing: you should always be well hydrated, but drinking a little more will cut down on the amount of sodium released during sweating. If this doesn't solve your problem, try petroleum jelly or runners lube to lesson the friction anywhere you experience it while running.

Your loose running clothes can also be a problem when trying to avoid chafing. The constant movement can cause your nipples to become irritated and even begin bleeding. Not only does this hurt, it can be embarrassing. Try wearing a snug-fitting singlet, which can help you avoid chafing and the discomfort that goes along with it.

Frostbite

When you head out the door for a long run in the dead of winter, remember to cover your hands and ears. I have lived and coached at high altitude for 20-plus years, so I'm constantly reminding my athletes to wear gloves and hats when the thermometer starts to dip, but it never fails that some freshman thinks he or she is tougher than old Mother Nature.

The extremities of your toes and feet, hands, ears, nose, and even penis are the most commonly frostbit areas. Covering these parts well is essential. You should take the precaution of selecting proper garments during colder weather. Layering clothes is also important to prevent hypothermia. If it's too cold to go outside, find a treadmill or cross-train that day.

Superficial frostbite is most recognizable by white or gray patches on the skin. The skin feels cold and stiff but is softer underneath the affected area. With this level of frostbite you should see a doctor if possible, but if that isn't possible, submerge the frostbitten area in warm water. Not *hot* water, as this could cause more problems. This warming up can take a half hour or more, but continue until your tissue softens.

If you happen to be out longer and get deep frostbite, the symptoms of this are waxy, pale skin, and sometimes blisters will occur. Seek medical attention immediately. Most runners will only get superficial frostbite, as your exposure to extreme cold usually isn't long enough to get deep frostbite.

Sunburn

You're out having a great run on a beautiful day and you don't have a care in the world. As you finish your run you look at your shoulders' red tint and feel a mild sting—ouch! Many times this is the extent of your sunburn, but it can be much worse. Long-term exposure to the sun increases your risk of skin cancer.

If you avoid using sunscreen because you don't like that sticky lotion feeling, try a lightweight lotion that is sweat-proof. You may like the feel of this lotion better, and you'll get the protection you need from the sun's rays.

Windburn

If you're out in extremely cold and windy conditions, you're likely to suffer from windburn. These conditions strip the body's natural oil from your skin, leaving it dried out and irritated. Your skin will look burned as with sunburn, but really all you need is to restore oil and moisture to the skin.

Your best protection for wind burn on the face is to grow a beard. If you're male and haven't started shaving yet or female and don't want to grow a beard, then there are other alternatives. The prevention techniques used for windburn and sunburn should go hand in hand: cover your skin, use sunscreen, and moisturize.

Also don't forget to use sunscreen in the winter. You don't realize you are receiving as many UV rays when it's cold outside. Sunscreen helps protect against UV rays as well as providing moisturizing agents to prevent windburn. Aloe-based moisturizers can also help alleviate the symptoms of windburn.

Dehydration and Heat Exhaustion

Running in the heat during the middle of summer raises several risks you certainly need to avoid. Dehydration most commonly means a bad performance for your workout or race, but continuing to run without rehydrating can lead to heat stroke and even death. Water is essential to all of your cells; your performance and health depend on your hydration habits.

It is not uncommon to lose a couple of pounds of water during an hour-long workout. Dehydration of 1 percent can decrease your running performance by 2 or 3 percent. Over a 10k, that can be as much as 1 to 2 minutes for a 45 minute run. You're at least going to have a horrible run, and if you're more than 3 percent dehydrated, you risk more serious problems.

Preventing dehydration is so much smarter than having to catch up. I see lots of athletes try to catch up on hydrating by trying to consume large quantities of water at one time. The problem is, once you're thirsty, you have already reached one stage of dehydration. It is imperative that you start every day and every run fully hydrated. It is best to drink water throughout the day, at least six to eight 8-ounce glasses of water a day at rest, as well as 5 to 7 ounces of water or electrolyte drink every for 15 minutes you run.

If you go for a long run, your body cannot absorb water at the same rate you sweat it out. On a hot run, you can lose as much as 3 to 5 pounds of water per hour. For runs that last longer than 45 minutes, you need to drink water about every 15 to 20 minutes. Use your water bottle to make this easier to accomplish and fully hydrate after your run.

If you run hard without proper hydration on a very hot day (90–100 degrees), you risk heat cramping and/or heat exhaustion. If you run hard on an extremely hot day (105–115 degrees and higher), you likely risk heat exhaustion or, worse, heat stroke. Take great precautions when running in hot weather: be sure to fully hydrate and continue hydrating through the run. Also run in the coolest part of the early morning or late evening to avoid the heat. Proper hydration will help you prevent heat exhaustion, however, when the heat index reaches 90-100 you should exercise caution. Anytime the heat index reaches greater than 100, consider an alternative workout.

Legs, Knees, Hips

Taking care of yourself from the waist down is vital to keeping you out on the track or the road.

Runner's Knee

Chondromalacia, usually known as runner's knee, is a common running injury that involves pain under the patella or kneecap. This injury is frequently caused by muscle imbalance; often the quadriceps is too tight and the hamstring too week, causing the kneecap to be pulled down. As the knee bends, the joint rubs away at the cartilage on the back of the kneecap, causing discomfort and swelling. It can actually wear away the back of the cartilage and rub it raw.

When chondromalacia strikes, you can take a NSAID or see your doctor for a stronger anti-inflammatory drug. Both will provide similar results, depending on the severity of your discomfort, but it's never a bad idea to see your doctor if you have any concerns.

Long term, you can alleviate chondromalacia by stretching the quadriceps, which will relax the muscle and restore balance. Massaging the quadriceps will also relax it. The next step is to strengthen the hamstring so there is better balance between the quad and hamstring muscles.

Here is an exercise that will help quell the pain. Sitting on the ground, put a pillow under your thigh behind your knee joint, then push your knee cap to the ground while lifting your foot. Repeat this 15 times as it will strengthen and relax your quadriceps and alleviate the pain.

Leg Cramps

There are two distinct theories of how and why leg cramping occurs. The first one deals with overexertion of a muscle to abnormal fatigue. The muscle recruitment/central nervous system malfunctions and can't release a full contraction, thus creating a painful cramp. The second theory deals with dehydration and electrolyte imbalances. The electrolytes that deal with muscle contractions and relaxation are potassium, calcium, magnesium, and sodium. Insufficient amounts of these electrolytes could be the source of your problem.

If you suffer from cramping in the legs, try one of the following remedies. When one of our runners has severe cramping, we prescribe massage—not your general feel-good massage, but rather a reconditioning of the muscle tissue. If you don't have or can't afford a masseuse, try massaging yourself with a foam roller or a stick-roller massager.

Calf muscles are especially susceptible to overuse injuries. You can ice and stretch injured calf and leg muscles, but be careful when stretching the calves; overstretching can slow recovery.

If your tightness continues and you have access to a physical therapist, try ultrasound or e-stim (electrical stimulation) treatments. I have found these to be valuable and effective treatments for tight muscles and strains.

Quad Tightness

Your quadriceps is the largest muscle in your upper thigh. Strains are common for this muscle, and I've found that it responds very well to specific treatments. Stretching and massage seem to get the best results, but we have also found great success with e-stim and ultrasound as well.

When the quad is injured to the point you can't run, try other activities until it heals. However, don't choose biking, as the quadriceps are the prime movers in biking, too. We do a lot of pool running, or swimming using only the upper body, allowing the quads more complete rest. Pool running allows the muscles to work without much resistance and is a good cardio workout for the whole body.

Shin Splints

If you have shin splints, welcome to the club, as this is one of the most common injuries with new and beginning runners. A sheath surrounds the bone and muscles that attach up and down your shin; if this muscle and sheath become too tight from swelling or overuse, the muscle and sheath can actually tear away from the bone. As you might imagine (or maybe you don't have to!), this is most painful.

Usually, this happens to runners who start with too much training or accelerate their training too quickly. You will need to spend time stretching this area of the leg as it often gets overlooked. If you do get shin splints, you definitely want to do some stretching and go heavy on the icing. Ignoring shin splints and allowing them to get aggravated can lead to an even worse injury, stress fractures.

But what should you do when you have shin splints? It is important that you try and catch this problem in the early stages. Cut back the volume and intensity of your training significantly, to allow your shins time to recover. Ice five to six times a day for 15 minutes and take an anti-inflammatory for a week to help reduce the swelling and prevent your problem from getting worse. If you have extremely tight muscles in your calves and shins, stretching and sports massage are likely to help.

Compartment Syndrome

It's important to watch for signs of compartment syndrome, a medical condition where increased pressure or swelling impairs the body's ability to transport blood.

Compartment syndrome is different from shin splints, which involves the muscle pulling away from the bone. With compartment syndrome, the muscle swells within its sheath. Because the connective tissues and sheaths that cover your muscles cannot stretch, the swelling and/or bleeding that occurs within the muscle tissues have no place to go.

Some types of compartment syndrome are caused by repetitive use of the muscles, such as running. Generally this does not result in an emergency, but it can in severe cases cause temporary or permanent damage to nerves and muscle tissue.

The signals generally are a pulse deficit, paralysis, or pain in the muscle compartment that won't go away. Seek medical attention immediately if you have an acute attack of compartment syndrome. Testing for compartment syndrome is done by checking the pressure inside your muscle compartments. The level of the pressure will help gauge the needed treatment.

Acute compartment syndrome is a medical emergency that requires immediate surgery to relieve the pressure within your muscle compartment. Treatment will involve rest, time off from running or exercise, anti-inflammatory medications, and stretching. If you have chronic compartment syndrome, address it; if left untreated, it can become acute and require more serious treatment.

IT Band

The iliotibial band, or IT band, is a muscle that runs from the hip, over the knee, and down into the ankle. When the IT band becomes overly tight, one cause is from running on the outside of your foot (suppination), so the pounding that your leg is taking is not being evenly distributed and your IT band is taking the brunt.

IT band problems can also arise if you are running on severely slanted roads in the same direction all the time. If you always run on the same side of the road—and this is usually the case because runners are creatures of habit—it puts more pressure on one leg, thus causing overuse and tightening of the IT band.

Road Blocks

IT band injuries can also happen if you buy shoes that are not made for your style of running.

As the IT band becomes extremely tight, it can worsen if not dealt with appropriately. One serious problem is when the IT band becomes very tight and gets inflamed and irritated at the knee joint. If your IT band is relaxed, it can slide over the knee joint easily, but when it is extremely tight it can catch on the nodule on the outside of the knee joint and become inflamed at this friction point. The IT band will start to snap over the nodule like a rubber band.

In Their Shoes

Kim was one dedicated college athlete, with a determination and tenacity that not many runners can muster. During her junior year cross-country season, she began to develop a slight pain (more like a tightness) in her front shin area. It felt like a muscle injury, but also had the warning signs of a stress fracture.

The pain gradually increased during our conference and regional cross-country meets. Although it hurt, she felt okay enough to keep running, and we took the necessary and usual steps to address it, including NSAIDS (nonsteroidal anti-inflammatory drugs), ice, and massage. The injury seemed to be responding.

Going into our national cross-country meet in Pomona, California, Kim's leg seemed better and we felt she would be okay. She got off to a good start in her race, but soon started to fall back. I made my way to the finish line, waiting for each of my athletes to finish. Kim was not near the front, which was unusual for her, a many-time All-American who'd even won a couple of national titles. I began to worry about her leg and the possibility of injury.

Finally the medical cart arrived; Kim was being transported by emergency personnel. She was in intense pain and we immediately took the ambulance to the hospital in Los Angeles, where physicians tried to figure out the problem. Eventually a specialist diagnosed compartment syndrome in Kim's lower leg. When the doctor did her initial evaluation, Kim had less than 5 percent blood flow going to her foot—her foot was not getting the oxygen it needed, and she was in jeopardy of losing her foot. The doctor immediately decided to operate.

Kim's surgery involved cutting the sheath that covered the muscles in her calf, which gave her muscles room to expand. After surgery, Kim's relief was almost immediate; the pressure was gone and normal blood flow had returned to her foot. Kim was out from running for nearly 10 weeks. Through rehab and careful planning, she slowly eased back into cross-training. Eventually, Kim returned to running and collegiate racing, where she continued her storied career.

Massage the larger part of the tendon midway between your knee and your hip. Massaging directly over the injury will only make the problem worse; only massage the uninjured part.

One treatment for this injury uses a 4- or 6-inch foam roller. Begin by laying the foam roller on the ground directly under your hip area. Then with all your weight distributed on both your elbow and the roller, pull or drag yourself across the roller until you reach just before the knee, and then push your body back to the original position. Repeat this exercise back and forth several times. This can leave you sore the first few times you do it, but you should continue it unless it becomes painful. As you build up some tolerance to this activity, you can increase the number of repetitions you do each day.

> **Watch Your Step**
>
> When you feel IT pain, you don't want to massage the band over the knee area because it is already inflamed.

Muscle Matters

Everyday aches and pains are part of the territory for runners. Sometimes they're more serious and require professional attention, but sometimes you just need to take some easy measures at home.

Muscle Imbalances

If you've been training hard, but maybe neglected some part of your total development training program, you may find yourself with muscle-imbalance problems. Your muscles can become tight and need extra stretching. The most frequently overlooked muscles are your hamstrings, calves, quadriceps, and hip flexors. And usually your weakest muscles are your glutes (butt), hip abductors and adductors, and abdominals.

Your posture and biomechanics will suffer greatly as a result of these imbalances, so if you want to increase your running performance and prevent injuries, you'll need to deal with them. If you're trying to develop that complete, well-rounded program to avoid these muscle imbalances, be sure your program includes flexibility and strength training, as well as balance and agility.

Muscle Pulls and Strains

All of the pulls and strains in this section are related to abdominal, calf, glutes, hamstring, piriformis, and psoas.

Muscle pulls and strains are caused by excessive stretching of the muscle fibers. Strains happen as a result of poor flexibility, low strength, muscle fatigue, improper balance between protagonist and antagonist muscles, and improper or insufficient warm-up.

Treatment of strains depends on the severity of the injury. If the injury is severe, I suggest you see a physician to prescribe your treatment. If it seems mild to moderate, begin with *RICE* therapy. Anti-inflammatory drugs will help alleviate swelling and pain. Once the pain and swelling have been reduced you should begin light stretching. If this goes well, try strengthening to rebuild the strength of the injured muscle.

Muscle Soreness and Tears

As you begin to step up your training, it's common to have some muscle soreness. For you beginning runners who go out for that 2- to 4-mile run then follow it up with some push-ups and sit-ups, you're bound to have some muscle soreness tomorrow or the next day. This is your body's natural way of dealing with unusual exertion and is part of the adjustment process that leads to greater endurance and strength. Muscle soreness is commonly at its nastiest within the first two days and begins to lessen over the next couple of days.

One important lesson you'll need to learn early in the process of getting fit is how you distinguish between "soreness" and "pain." Delayed-onset muscle soreness (DOMS) usually occurs between a few hours and a next day or two after the exercise is completed. This is very different from the acute pain that comes from pulling or straining a muscle. If you suffer a severe muscle strain or tear, you will feel it immediately; this type of pain often has swelling and/or bruising associated with it.

Muscle soreness can be a result of very small tears of the muscle tissue. The quantity of tears (and soreness) will certainly depend on how tough and extensive your exercise was. Running and other exercises that cause your muscles to forcefully contract and lengthen cause the most tenderness. The type of running and exercising that seems to get you the most would include bounding (plyometrics), running downhill, weight training (with emphasis on the downward action), or squats, push-ups, and dips.

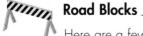

Road Blocks

Here are a few tips to dealing with muscle soreness:

- Time is the number-one healer. Your muscle soreness will generally go away in a few days.
- If you're extremely sore, don't overdue it.
- Submerging sore muscles in ice is a great way to decrease that inflammation.
- Mild stretching works.
- Gently massage the effected muscle.
- Try an anti-inflammatory (ibuprofen).
- Utilize a proper warm-up and cool down.

If you do happen to have a muscle tear you will surely know it. If so, then you will need to put some ice and compression on the area quickly. The sooner you do this, the better, as you can shorten your recovery time by not letting the injury swell. See a physician to make sure you're handling your healthy return to running properly.

PMS

Premenstrual Syndrome (PMS) is described as the physical and psychological changes that females have prior to their periods. PMS can cause mild to severe physical discomfort as well as emotional distress. The symptoms of PMS can include swollen breasts, headaches, fatigue, dizziness, stomach cramps and bloating, backaches, fluid retention, weight gain, mood swings, and depression.

PMS symptoms tend to vanish or greatly improve once bleeding actually starts. Running can relieve the symptoms of PMS; that runner's high that you get after running may help you fight the depression and mood swings.

However, female runners' monthly loss of blood increases their likelihood of becoming anemic. Both men and women who run have larger requirements for iron; running produces larger amounts of red blood cells, which increases your need for additional iron. As a runner you will take thousands of footsteps on your daily runs, which causes damage to your red blood cells that can lead to iron loss and anemia.

Your iron stores can also be depleted by the increased sweating you're having as a result of long endurance running. Profuse sweating can increases your risk of becoming anemic. Being iron deficient can create a multitude of problems for your running performance as well as your overall health, if you have any of these risk factors, you should probably be supplementing iron. Consult your physician about iron supplementation; this will help you avoid the woes of anemia.

Stress Reaction and Fractures

Stress fractures account for nearly 10 percent of all athletic-related injuries. These stress fractures are most commonly seen in runners, but do occur in other athletes as well. It is interesting to note that nearly all (95 percent) stress fractures occur in your lower half of your body.

A stress fracture is one of the worst injuries a runner can suffer. It's not a complete break, it's a hairline fracture. There's not much you can do to rehab it except allow four to eight weeks for it to heal. In severe cases it won't heal properly because of chronic trauma or poor nutrition, in which case the down time can last three to five months, although this is not typical.

Stress fractures typically occur in your weight-bearing bones, such as the tibia and fibula in the lower leg and the metatarsals in the foot.

Stress fractures don't have a lot of symptoms, but the pain can be excruciating. New stress fractures often won't show up on x-rays; it usually takes a couple weeks for them to be seen. Bone scans are most effective in showing new stress fractures. Check with your insurance company to see if these x-rays are covered in your policy before getting one—they can be expensive.

Typically you'll have a generalized area of pain that includes tenderness and is most painful when you put weight on it. Also, as you run, your stress fracture may start out very painfully, lessen to some degree, and then be excruciating to severe by the end.

With stress fractures, you're looking at stationary bike riding or other nonweight-bearing exercises for rehab. I have found that the pool is excellent for cross-training with a stress fracture. Swimming allows you to get completely off those legs and work hard on your cardiovascular system.

Trocanteric Bursitis

This injury is common with long endurance runners. If you feel pain between your upper femur and the muscles located in that area, you probably have bursitis. The pain is caused by inflammation in one or two of the bursae sacs located there. Your pain will usually stay in the area of your upper outer thigh. Continuing to run on this injury will irritate the bursae sacs, thus increasing the pain.

The normal treatment begins with the RICE method, which is a good course for many injuries. Anti-inflammatory drugs are also effective when dealing with bursitis. If these methods do not alleviate the fluid, swelling, and associated pain, have a doctor drain the fluid from the bursae sacs.

The Least You Need to Know

- The elements—sun or frost—are foes, not friends.
- Skin irritations can actually force you off track.
- Back pain is not usually related to running, but it can be aggravated by running.
- You can treat muscle strains without letting them slow you down.

Chapter 15

Finding the Right Medical Care

In This Chapter

◆ Why you shouldn't avoid medical help

◆ How to find the right care for you

◆ Some options outside of the mainstream

◆ Taking time off to start with

Okay, it's time to seek the services and support of the medical community to get you back on track. Different types of medical professionals may be able to provide the care you require. A major consideration before seeking care from any of these providers is to determine the provider's philosophy and experience with sports medicine and/or injury recovery.

What's a Running Doctor?

When people use the term "sports medicine," they are referring to an interdisciplinary team of medical professionals who focus on the treatment and preventive care of athletes. This team can often include physicians, surgeons, physical therapists, athletic trainers, coaching staff—and, of course, the athlete. If you aren't blessed with your own personal entourage of care providers, I will try to provide some basic information on the medical care that *is* available to you. Picking the right provider for your needs will cut down on your lost time.

It's important to determine whether the provider is sports or injury focused. Too often, you might seek care from a provider who tells you to "take six weeks off and call me if it doesn't feel better." This might be required for some types of injuries or conditions, but most times a sports-injury specialist can help you develop a broader plan that will address your condition and still keep you working toward your fitness or racing goals.

Sports medicine doctors work specifically with sports injuries. They are physicians who finish a primary residency program, then obtain one to two years of additional training through a fellowship in sports medicine. Their focus is on the treatment of injuries related to sports and activities, but also on prevention. They have focused knowledge on the effects of training and competition. This is a growing field in medicine, but it's fairly new and not available everywhere.

A family physician, family practitioner, or general practitioner usually sees patients of all ages and both sexes for both outpatient and inpatient work. Their training is broad and covers many conditions, injuries, or situations. The scope of services in each office will vary. Some family doctors have an inclination toward sports medicine and can help get you back to training. If you need specialized care, they are a great source for specialists or treatments that might work for you.

Podiatrists specialize in disorders of the ankle and the foot, sometimes providing care for the knee, leg, hips, and all lower extremities. Their scope of services vary from state to state. Some doctors of podiatric medicine do surgery; others may limit their care to outpatient medicine. Be sure you understand the services available as you select the right podiatrist.

Radiologists specialize in using medical imaging technology to diagnose and sometimes treat disease. The most common applications used in injury detection are basic x-ray, computed tomography (CT), or magnetic resonance imaging (MRI). Each of these tools is useful in figuring out an injury; your doctor can decide which one to use for which injury.

A regular x-ray machine directs radiation upon a specific portion of the body. The denser materials such as bone absorb the radiation differently than skin, fat, or muscle, which helps create an image that providers can use to see a potential broken bone or other injury. CT scanning adds another dimension to the imagining process and often will show finer details. MRI has become an essential diagnostic tool, giving the best soft-tissue contrast. It does require that patients hold still for extended periods, but even this has improved. More and more athletes nowadays get MRIs to diagnose bone injury and possible stress fractures.

A doctor of orthopedic surgery specializes in a branch of surgery focused on the musculoskeletal system. These doctors treat trauma as well as acute, chronic, and overuse injuries, using both surgical and nonsurgical strategies. An orthopedic physician may have an area of focus beyond orthopedic surgery ranging from surgical sports medicine, to joint reconstruction, to a foot and ankle focus.

The use of arthroscopic instruments has been of great value for injured athletes. Often this treatment will allow a less invasive procedure and shorten the recovery period. This has become one of the most common operations performed by orthopedic surgeons and can get some runners back to training after a short recovery period.

Exclusively for Her

Female athletes face unique challenges to keep their bodies healthy and fit, and their doctor of obstetrics and gynecology (OB/GYN) can help. Sometimes a training program can interrupt the menstrual cycle or cause other women's health concerns. The lack of a menstrual cycle can keep you from producing the necessary components needed to keep your bones strong and injury-free.

Runners who are pregnant need to consult with their physician about their training regiment. While in most cases it is okay and even encouraged to keep training during pregnancy, it is imperative to involve your physician in this conversation. They can assist you in adjusting volume and intensity and give you guidance on an adequate recovery period for your personal condition.

‍rainers

‍‍‍‍‍‍ therapy is a great complement to other types of medical care. It is designed to develop, maintain, and restore maximum movement and function. Some common conditions that physical therapists treat are back and neck pain, biomechanical problems, muscular control issues, and all types of sports-related injuries.

Therapists generally work with you to set out a treatment plan that can involve as few as two or three visits to as many as several visits per week. Their treatments often include movement enhancement, functional training, electrotherapeutic and mechanical treatments and procedures, not to mention patient education and instruction.

I have also found that massage therapy is helpful in injury recovery when combined with other therapeutic treatments. It stimulates the muscles and relieves stress and tightness. I often incorporate massage, or rubdowns if you're in the gym, into my training programs. It is a great way to do some injury prevention with your muscles and can help you return after an injury.

At Adams State College, we rely heavily on athletic trainers who specialize in the prevention, evaluation, treatment, and management of injuries or illness, including rehabilitation. These professionals are highly involved in the day-to-day training of both professional and amateur athletes, prepping athletes for practice and competition, and evaluating injuries to outline a treatment course.

While most of us think of athletic trainers as being on the sidelines in everything from high-school games to professional football playoffs, there are often athletic trainers at local health clubs, industrial settings, military facilities, and sports medicine programs. Hospitals and outpatient medical settings can also incorporate athletic trainers into their services.

Diet Doctors

Looking for some advice on your diet? Or maybe you have a chronic medical condition that merits some evaluation of your health and nutrition? A nutrition specialist can give you advice on dietary matters.

Nutritionists can have varying levels of degrees, backgrounds, and experience. It is not a legally protected term, so the credibility of the person isn't guaranteed. You may hear or read dietary and nutrition advice from people calling themselves nutritionists, but it may not be sound advice from a licensed professional.

I suggest using a registered dietitian (RD), a professional registered with the American Dietetic Association. They are only able to use the label "dietician" when they have met strict, specific educational requirements and passed a national exam.

Don't Underestimate the Power of the Mind

A sports psychologist has received special training in behavior related to sports and competition. He or she usually has education in exercise science and physical education as well as training in psychology and counseling.

Runners can be intense—we can be compulsive, and when our injuries prevent us from working out or working out at the level we are accustomed to, we occasionally need help adjusting. Sometimes you may need help understanding the psychological/mental factors affecting your performance. A sports psychologist can help you manage your emotions related to your injury and work with you to develop coping skills as you recover.

Sports counseling can be helpful in competition performance and goal setting as well. Some important skills taught by sports psychologists are relaxation, visualization, positive self-talk, emotion control, concentration, and periodization in training. Many of these principles also work well with other movement activities, public speaking, or music performance.

A Few Alternative Types of Care

Chiropractic care is the alternative health-care profession whose purpose is diagnosing and treating mechanical disorders of the spine and musculoskeletal system to affect the nervous system and improve health. Chiropractors use a variety of treatments to address a variety of patient concerns. The most common treatment is spinal adjustment, which attempts to properly adjust the spine and allow the nerves to do their job better.

Some chiropractors specialize in sports injuries or specific musculoskeletal problems. They can combine traditional treatments with nutrition or exercises to increase spinal strength and improve overall health. Chiropractors do not prescribe drugs, and see their role as providing a drug-free alternative treatment plan.

Active release therapy (ART) treats injuries related to muscle overuse. It uses patented soft-tissue and movement-based massage to treat problems with muscles, tendons, ligaments, fascia, and nerves. The provider uses touch and massage to address the injury by evaluating texture, tightness, and movement (or lack of it) in a specific body area. It isn't a standardized treatment; it's focused on the individual. Several of my athletes have benefited from ART, and it can be helpful in treating joint pain, sciatica, plantar fasciitis, and shin splints.

Acupuncture is the technique of inserting and manipulating needles into points on the body to unblock chi and balance-opposing forces. According to acupuncture theory, this will assist in restoring health and well-being and has particular benefits in the area of pain relief. The body is treated as a whole that involves functional systems loosely associated with physical organs. Disease and injury are interpreted as the loss of balance between yin and yang, and the treatments seek to restore that balance.

The Least You Need to Know

◆ Finding the right doctor is as important as having the right shoes.

◆ Alternative treatments can be effective.

◆ Getting help with your diet can accelerate gains.

◆ Massages feel great and have great healing power.

Chapter 16

Running with Injury and Illness

In This Chapter

- ◆ How to recognize an injury
- ◆ When you will get back up to speed after resuming training
- ◆ What amount of time allows small injuries to heal
- ◆ When anti-inflammatories might be dangerous

This chapter will give you the same advice I give my athletes about what is an acceptable amount of pain and/or soreness. I'll also explain the pitfalls of continuing when you shouldn't. Most runners—nearly 70 percent, in fact—will have to take time off because of an injury, so you're not alone.

Soreness and Pain

It's important that you learn the difference between soreness and pain. Sometimes extreme soreness can be just as aggravating as an injury, but soreness will eventually disappear, while an injury seems to linger forever.

Answering the following questions will help you determine if you're injured or just extremely sore:

◆ Did your pain come on gradually or did it seem to pop up out of thin air?

◆ Can you explain why you're having pain or soreness?

◆ Was it a particular workout that you did today or yesterday?

◆ Did you step in a hole or slightly twist an ankle that you thought nothing of when it happened?

◆ Have you been increasing your mileage without thought of proper periodization?

These questions can help you determine whether your injury is acute or chronic and whether you can train through it.

Pain: Stage 1

The pain you get from running usually follows a series of stages, unless it is an acute injury, in which case you probably know how it happened because your pain was immediate. During the first stage, you probably won't feel much pain until your run is finished, and even then you may not describe it as significant pain, more like tightness or discomfort.

This type of pain or discomfort will seem to fade away as you start to run the next day, but will seem just a hair worse that evening or the next morning when you roll out of bed. This process can continue for a couple of days or a week, until one morning the pain is so much worse you wonder why you waited until now to do something about it.

If you're in this situation, remember: "When in doubt, don't." The smart thing to do in stage 1 is to stop running for one to two days, receive treatment, and try to eliminate the cause of this pain and not just the symptoms. Taking time off when you need it (now) will serve you best in the long haul and will allow you more running days later.

If you feel that you must continue to run, you should at least cut back your mileage by half, which should be enough of a reduction to allow the injury to properly heal while continuing running. If the injury still doesn't seem to be getting any better, you should definitely take two or three days off from running.

I typically tell my athletes to attack an injury with the shotgun approach versus the BB gun approach. I've seen many doctors and athletic trainers give runners very conservative advice and treatment, but I've had great success dealing with injuries very aggressively from the get-go. I have my runners ice 6 to 10 times a day (10 minutes every hour). This will stop any bleeding of damaged tissues and will promote healing after you finish icing as the blood rushes to rewarm the injury. I also have runners use compression and elevation, receive massages, and take NSAIDs (over-the-counter nonsteroidical anti-inflammatory drugs such as ibuprofen). All of these can shorten the length of the injury.

Sometimes you won't know what healed the injury because you used so many treatments at once, but who cares? You're healed and can get back out on the road. Many times a doctor or athletic trainer will start you icing for a few days, then move to the next therapy if that doesn't work—a process that could take a week or more when maybe you could have been back out there in one or two days.

Pain: Stage 2

If your injury has progressed to the second stage, you've probably noticed some discomfort during your run. It hasn't yet turned to pain, and you still feel up to running and can manage hard workouts and races, but you can sometimes feel tightness and soreness while running.

This is the critical time to use a commonsense approach; you don't want to roll the dice and keep running without regard to these warning signs (the odds aren't good). Speaking from 27 years of experience, the commonsense approach will serve you well. Take two to three days completely off from running and receive treatments (rest, ice, compression, elevation, NSAIDs, plus your physical therapist may prescribe e-stim or ultrasound). If you treat the injury properly, you can completely wipe out the pain and continue injury-free running.

Pain: Stage 3

If you've ignored the discomfort and it has progressed into pain while you run, and you feel like the only way to get better is to back off or stop running completely, then you've reached the third stage. This stage will definitely take a longer time to recover from. Typically you will need to take one to four weeks to fully recover, with 5 to 10 days off from running.

You can still cross-train, and I recommended it as long as it doesn't aggravate your injury. However, many injuries can be exacerbated by cross-training, so be careful and use your time off from running to stay fit but also to fully recuperate.

You should follow the treatments in stages 1 and 2, and you can most definitely benefit from e-stim and/or ultrasound. See a physical therapist or athletic trainer for rehab and strengthening exercises before you return to running. This will help you steer clear of any reoccurrences or new injuries.

Pain: Stage 4

If you ignored the warning signs and let yourself progress to the fourth stage, then you have stopped running as the pain has become too severe. This has turned into a chronic overuse injury. Most likely you're going to miss three to six weeks of running, and even the shorter time period will require lots of therapy and TLC.

It is very important to receive therapy and complete it even when you are taking time off from running. I've seen runners take three to four weeks off from this type of injury and not do any therapy, then try to run, thinking they should be completely healed, only to be shocked that the injury seems just as bad. With the type of injury you have now, I advise seeing a sports doctor or a specialist if at all possible, as he or she may be able to prescribe a stronger anti-inflammatory and more aggressive treatments that may lessen your time off.

Listen to Your Pain

Pain is very important to listen to; it's your warning that something is wrong. Pay extra attention to any bone pains that you may have, as the recovery is long with stress reactions and stress fractures. If you have bone pain, take *immediate* time off until this sensation goes away. This type of injury can progress very quickly once you start to feel it.

Taking NSAIDs is a definite no-no with bone pain, as they can mask the pain until you have a full-blown stress fracture. If you're just starting to feel the pain, an x-ray probably won't show the injury. If you catch this injury early enough, you may only need to take a week or two off; if you let it go for another week or two, you may be facing a six- to eight-week layoff.

Most runners' injuries are a result of overuse and occur over a period of time, so they won't go away in just a day or two. Normally it will take about the same amount of time as the time you have run with this injury to completely rid yourself of all the symptoms—and that's *if* you complete all your treatments.

The most important thing is to catch the injury early and "shoot it with the shotgun" (get as much treatment as possible). This will limit your shelf time and get you back on the road as quickly as possible. When you're in doubt about the nature and severity of your injury, a couple easy or completely off days now can prevent stage 4 and a mandatory four- to six-week time out.

Running with Illness

In spite of our healthy pursuit of fitness, most runners tend to ignore the warning signs of illness just as much as injuries. I will share with you the same advice that I give to my team when they're sick.

Training Your Immune System

If you're running for health and fitness and run 3 to 4 miles a day, three to four times per week, then this type of exercise actually strengthens your immune system. But if you're running to improve racing times and training more than 40 miles per week—even up to 80 or 90 miles a week—then you significantly increase your risk of injury and illnesses.

Running high-intensity workouts and high mileage for extended periods can overstress your immune system and weaken it, allowing viral infections to flourish. Most American distance runners get two or three infections a year, which can become a significant factor in your overall training program.

If you choose a higher-mileage program, consider taking supplements to keep your immune system strong. You should also consider getting a flu shot as you will be more at risk for these type infections. I typically like my athletes to receive the flu shot, as it is good preventative medicine, and getting the flu is an automatic few days off from running.

Runner Facts

Here are a few signs that your immune system may be low:

- ◆ Fatigue that is beyond normal
- ◆ Need increased recovery time from intervals or from hard day to hard day
- ◆ Seem to catch colds and the flu more frequently
- ◆ Insomnia
- ◆ Complete exhaustion after normal training workouts

Over the years, I have found that many of my runners who are vegetarians have a higher incidence of colds and infections. Amino acids can help counteract the effects of free radicals produced during metabolism (the chemical reaction that happens in your cells to convert food into the energy) that can disrupt our cells from working properly.

If your immune system is low and you're catching every cold possible, you may want to increase your intake of vitamins A, C, and E. These vitamins help to regulate the number of T cells you produce; T cells help the immune system respond to infections. The minerals selenium and zinc also help stimulate the immune system. With the exception of selenium, these are all better ingested as a part of your regular diet than as supplements. Selenium is not readily available in the foods we eat; therefore it should be taken as a supplement.

To Run or Not to Run?

That is the question. What are the signs to look for? First of all, if you're even asking this question, the answer is probably no, but some colds are mild enough that we can push through without any adverse effects. As always, use caution when in doubt. Following is a more in-depth look at the most common illnesses runners face, and how you might determine whether you should or shouldn't run in each case.

If you've got an ordinary head cold with the usual symptoms, you can continue to run. However, you should realize that you're probably not going to feel that great while running. You should also cut back your volume and intensity to ensure that the cold doesn't move into your lungs. If the infection does move into your lungs, you should be more careful, as this can delay your return to running.

If you have a persistent sore throat, consult your physician, as you may have strep, which should be treated with antibiotics (make sure you take them all). Strep can get much worse if left untreated. If any of your cold symptoms persist or worsen, take a day or two off until you feel better and don't restart running until you feel better for a full 24 hours.

The flu is more complicated to run with, as the symptoms are much worse than the common cold. Two of the bigger problems with running with the flu are fever and dehydration, which can actually make running dangerous. Never run with a fever, as this will increase your risk of heat stroke and brain damage. Even after the flu is gone, use caution to prevent a relapse. The flu will usually leave you feeling low on energy, so start off slow in your return to running.

 Watch Your Step _____

A list of suggestions to protect you from injury and illness:

- Monitor your basal heart rate; if it is 15 percent higher than normal, take an easy day or a complete day off.
- Get plenty of sleep (8–9 hours).
- Don't train too many hard days in a given week.
- Avoid exposure to sick people.
- Wash your hands and keep hands away from face.
- Avoid losing too much weight too quickly.
- Eat a well-balanced diet that includes vitamins A, C, and E.
- Reduce stress from your lifestyle as much as possible.

If you get mononucleosis (mono), you will definitely need to sit out an extended period of time. Mono usually effects younger runners, but can be contracted by older runners as well. The greatest risk of running with mono is the potential of rupturing your spleen, which can be fatal. (It's certainly not worth the risk.) You will also delay your recovery by trying to train through this ailment; the recovery from mono can vary from person to person, but you'll usually need 6 to 10 weeks off from any hard physical activity.

Many illnesses have warning signs. Sometimes it's just a runny, stuffy nose, the first sign of overtraining in some runners. Others may seem to have constant nagging injuries like plantar fasciitis or Achilles tendonitis—classic warning signs that you are overtraining, usually followed by more severe injuries or illnesses. So pay attention to your body and the way it feels, as this is your first line of defense against injury and illness.

Healing on the Go: Cross-Training

You can still make gains when you can't run. There are times when you need to change up your training to get to your goal. When you have an injury or feel an injury creeping up, cross-training can provide valuable workouts and keep your fitness at a desired level.

Another important consideration is if you are the type of runner that needs some diversity in your training program or could benefit from additional improved muscle balance. Cross-training will help you build a different muscles than traditional running and give you added leg strength and muscle balance. This is especially important if you suffer from poor posture or other aches and pains associated with imbalanced muscles.

Giving Your System a Boost

You may find that you need to increase your volume of aerobic exercise, but your body isn't ready for the impact of additional running. Cross-training can give you these precious added minutes without the increased risk of overuse or impact injuries. The additional training will increase the size of your heart, which adds to your body's ability to handle increased blood flow; the increased blood flow will add to your ability to tolerate lactic acid, and ... you get the point. It can help!

Cross-training means something different to everyone who hears it. I use the term to mean training that is generally equivalent to the work effort that you would expend if you were running. If I suggest an activity that doesn't take the same type of effort, I call that complementary training.

It's important to know if you need or want your cross-training to involve weight-bearing or nonweight-bearing exercise. Do you want your legs and body to feel the impact of the exercise (treadmill or stair climber), or does your body need relief from such impact (swimming or biking)? All of these activities are great for cross-training, but different needs (or injuries) require different exercises.

If your cross-training is a recovery activity, such as when you have shin splints or a knee injury, then nonweight-bearing is your best bet. Use the bicycle or pool as your main venue. But if you're attempting to add some diversity into the workout routine, then traditional impact activities are fine.

Cross-Training Activities to Consider

Swimming is one of the best cross-training activities available. It's a great cardiovascular exercise. Although you can't get your heart rate as high as you do when running, you are still getting a great cardiovascular workout and keeping your legs off the road. Swimming is also great for building your upper body muscles and strength.

Another great water activity is deep-water running. It's exactly like it sounds. Using some type of flotation device (I suggest a flotation belt), you jump into the deep end and start running. Do the motions exactly like you were running down the road, and you will be amazed at how fast you feel the effects. Like swimming, there is no shock or impact on the legs. Both of these are great for recovering from an injury or just for some workout diversity.

If you're a really good swimmer and want to add an additional challenge to deep-water running, try doing it without a flotation device. Be sure to stay close to the edge and have someone keep an eye on you till you get the hang of it.

Get Out on the Bike

Cycling—riding a bicycle—can be a great cross-training workout. It allows you to work your quadriceps and shins at a higher intensity than these muscles usually get when you run. Both of these muscles are slower to develop than calves and hamstrings, so cycling can provide good muscle-balance benefits as well.

Cycling can be very similar to running in regards to how the efforts tax your body, so this isn't what you want to do for an easy day unless you adjust the intensity. I suggest cycling for the same amount of time that you had planned to run and let the distance take you where it may. Another added benefit of cycling is that you can cover more miles in the same amount of time as running, which can give you a few new views and add some spice to your training.

> **Watch Your Step**
>
> Safety first: if you get on a bike, always wear a helmet and ride with traffic. Cycling has its own set of rules, so know them and stay safe.

But cycling has a few risks as well. It usually requires that you ride on the road (unless you're lucky enough to live where trails are common), and, if the weather is not your friend, then cycling will be your enemy. Wet roads or windy conditions can quickly take the fun out of any new views that you might have encountered.

Skiing the Great Indoors

One of the great benefits of living in Colorado is the abundance of outdoor activities. Cross-country skiing is a great workout that builds cardiovascular fitness and strengthens both upper and lower body muscles. It's great for clearing the mind as well. There is nothing like a ski workout through a pristine mountain trail to build both your muscles and your spirit.

If you can't do real skiing, then a NordicTrack ski simulator machine works much the same way. It provides a challenging workout without the traditional leg pounding that running hands you.

If you are looking for a cross-training activity that builds hips, buttocks, and upper-body muscles, a rowing machine can be just the thing. It provides a strenuous workout without any pounding. It can be challenging to maintain your focus while rowing, but it will add some variety.

Both treadmills and stair-stepping machines are great alternative training choices, but it's important to remember that both of these do the same type of pounding on your legs and body as running down the road. I recommend both for adding diversity in your training, but this is not what you should do when you're trying to either rest your legs or recover from a pounding or overuse injury.

Sports You Might Not Think Of

There are many, many types of exercise and workouts that can benefit you. Some runners like to rollerblade; others love racquetball. I'm sure these exercises help your overall fitness, but they're not good substitutes for aerobic workouts, nor are they the equivalent of a run.

I suggest that if you love doing something and it improves your physical fitness, then do it. But bring it into your workout program on your traditionally easy days, to make sure that you don't lose overall fitness.

How Much Is Enough?

Die-hard runners will always struggle to see how cross-training will fit into their overall fitness programs. Too often, they won't know how to adjust or adapt this type of training into their schedule. They'll do too much or too little and end up setting themselves back.

Here is how you can figure out exactly how much to do. Convert the running workout for that day into time, then apply that time to your cross-training. If you were going to run 5 miles, but instead wanted to swim, figure out how long a 5-mile run would take and then swim for that period of time. Just like with running, add time for warming up and cooling down.

You can also convert running mileage to cross-training time: take your average pace per mile times the number of miles run (5 miles times 8 minutes per mile = 40 minutes of cross-training, plus 5 minutes for warm-up and 5 minutes for cooldown = 50 minutes of total cross-training time).

The same formula will work for cycling. If you're due for a long Sunday run, just convert it to time and set out on your bike. If you are due for a higher-intensity day, then adjust the same way. If you had planned to do an interval workout where you ran for 400 meters times 10, then figure out how long each 400 would take you and increase your intensity in the cross-training activity for the same period. Again, remember to warm up and cool down. Your body needs both to get ready for and recover from cross-training, just like your normal run.

> **Watch Your Step**
>
> You need to know that when doing nonweight-bearing activity, it's hard to get your heart rate as high as your target level, and your recovery heart rate drops faster as well.

Remember, if you've had an injury or illness, it is important to build volume before intensity. Your body will need to adapt to running again with low levels of stress. As it adapts, add more volume, then add intensity to help you prevent any reoccurrences.

The Least You Need to Know

- Pay attention to warning signs.

- Some illnesses, like the flu and mono, can't be "trained through."

- Don't expect your best times when you first start training again.

- Training too much taxes the immune system.

- Just because you can't run doesn't mean you stop training. Cycling, skiing machines, and rowers can help your aerobic base, and probably the safest cross-training activity is swimming.

Chapter 17

Staying Motivated

In This Chapter

- ◆ Why you have to stay upbeat
- ◆ How positive energy helps you stay healthy
- ◆ Why running can and should be fun
- ◆ Why running is a lifelong pursuit and passion

Over the years, I have taken great pride in ensuring that my teams were excited and motivated to start their training as well as their competitive seasons. I feel the key to success is maintaining a high level of motivation until our goals are met.

However, there are always distractions, injuries, and illnesses that can make you lose sight of your pursuit, so staying motivated is easier said than done.

The First Step Is the Most Important

As a coach at a very diverse state university, I work with runners from different geographical, economic, and sociological backgrounds. Although motivation comes from all different angles for these athletes, a few common threads allow many of them to achieve great success.

One of my favorite quotes I use often is attributed to Arthur Ashe: "Success is a journey, not a destination." I love this quote because it speaks to the long haul, not just the present. If we are to have any success, we must start the journey. So many runners tend to focus on the outcome and not the process. Staying motivated and continuing the journey creates the proper foundation for reaching injury-free success.

A great quote from Confucius is: "A journey of a thousand miles begins with a single step." Taking that first step can be your commitment to a new way of doing things, whether you're beginning running or just living a healthier lifestyle. After you take that first step, the next step is easier.

When you begin a running program or start back from an injury, the hardest part is getting going and staying with it long enough to realize your potential and your personal goals. The first few weeks of any new or returning training regimen takes a toll on you. You are sore and tired, and getting down on yourself seems easier than staying focused. At times like this, I believe it's essential to take a few minutes each day to remind yourself why you needed or wanted to do this.

The Value Factor

The value factor is one of the most important elements of motivation. If you are going to do anything, especially hard exercise like running, you have to believe you're going to benefit. I always ask my athletes, "If I could guarantee that if you worked your butts off—and I mean a *lot* of work—you would win a national title, would you do it?" Without any hesitation, they say, "Coach, if you guarantee it, I'll do whatever it takes." Then I tell them that the only guarantee is that if they *don't* work their butts off, they're certain *not* to win a national title!

For the value factor to really work, it needs to be strong enough to inspire each of us even in the face of adversity and injury. Life can be cruel, so it's important to develop a strong spirit and inner strength.

Runner Facts _____

Get to know the runners around you. This will help you understand where you fit on the performance curve and give you something to shoot for. I have a friend who is new to running. To stay injury-free in his first race, his personal goal was "to be in the top three of the old people who just run for fun." There's always a way to put a positive spin on staying injury-free!

If you're currently injured and have been for a while, then your motivation is probably suffering. It is important that you understand and focus on the value factor, in this case the long-term benefits of running, so you will keep up your cross-training or therapy and get back on the road as quickly as possible. Keeping up some type of training will keep you fit while you're getting healthy; it can also keep you from getting depressed. Staying motivated through the rough patches will make your later successes that much sweeter.

I know many runners who started running and stayed motivated because they value the self-improvement qualities associated with running. These qualities include looking good, losing weight, feeling better, and eating a more healthy diet, which are all splendid reasons to run. You should always be proud of yourself after you run: you've done something positive for your health and well-being! Make a mental note to reward yourself every so often—maybe have that dessert you've been craving—for your consistent, healthy lifestyle. Don't forget to be proud of yourself: it's a big part of keeping up your motivation.

Many of you may appreciate the stress-reduction benefits of running; these easy, long runs are great for that. I have gone on many runs where it seemed the pressures of work or other troubling experiences were washed away as the run progressed. This is another great benefit of running. I make it a point with my

Road Blocks _____

Don't get carried away in your first run or your first race and end up hurting yourself. Start slow and steady. If you still feel good as the race progresses, then keep moving up.

athletes to keep all the negative influences and negative talk away from practice. This should be a time to either work hard or enjoy, and both are much easier with a positive attitude.

Running provides so many great benefits; one that is often overlooked is the prevention of disease. If you run enough to raise your VO2 Max to 50 milliliters, you reduce the chance of cancer and cardiovascular disease to the smallest degree. If it's that simple, why aren't more people out running away from cancer and cardiovascular disease?

Positive Perspective Helps Overcome (and Prevent) Injuries

Mom and Dad used to always say, "If it was easy, then everyone could do it." Let this inspire you to think that you are not average and that you have what it takes to get through injuries and stay positive. If you love to run, you may or may not look forward to your cross-training, but stay positive and focus on the benefits you reap from this exercise. I know this is not always easy, but it's very rewarding to keep going when others can't or won't. (Remember: not everyone can, or they would!)

Overcoming obstacles like injuries certainly can make you a stronger person. I'm not suggesting that you go crazy with your training or cross-training; rather, that you have a mindset that this is something that you want to do because you value it. Whatever your reasons are, if they're strong enough, then you have a great chance of reaching your goals. If your motivations are strong enough, you'll do all the ancillary things that keep you healthy and fit, such as warming up and cooling down properly, hydrating well, getting enough sleep, taking necessary vitamins and supplements, and so on.

Obsessive Types: Too Much Is Too Much

Once you're motivated, though, it's important to manage yourself. I have to constantly hold back some athletes who always want to do more. Some runners tend to let their motivation get in the way of common sense, which usually ends up in injury or illness. Be cautious if you are an obsessive-compulsive person; I have many runners who have wrestled with this disorder. Obsessive-compulsive runners tend to be highly motivated and start doing extra workouts and training just for the sake of doing them.

Your motivation can sometimes exceed your fitness level, so you have to stay in control. Know yourself and the reasons you run. Make sure that your decision to run or not is based solely on your well-being and self-improvement. Enjoy the time you have to run. In our fast-paced society, we rarely take time to enjoy ourselves, and running can allow those rare moments. There are times when you run that you can let your mind wander and just enjoy the action of running.

On the other hand, I have some athletes who are always searching for a better reason to run. The old one just isn't strong enough to justify their efforts. These runners tend not to get excited about running because they are not achieving success. This brings us to the chicken or egg theory. Which comes first? Part of our motivation will come from achieving success, however big or small. But we have to put in quality work before we can have success. Once this process begins working right, running becomes like a powerful drug with addictive properties.

Intrinsic vs. Extrinsic

Where does your motivation come from? Is it easy to find? Sports psychologists talk in terms of intrinsic and extrinsic motivation. If you are motivated by a dangling carrot (prize money, trophies), then you are extrinsically motivated. If you're motivated by the drive to get better and improve your capabilities, then you are intrinsically motivated. Both are very powerful, but people who are intrinsically motivated tend to stay that way more consistently.

I teach my athletes that, once they become knowledgeable, they are responsible for achieving or not achieving their goals by the choices they make each day to either do or not do the entire program. This includes doing things the right way. I am a firm believer in doing things the right way. Shortcuts are the short path to injury and illness.

In Their Shoes

Intrinsic versus extrinsic motivation is always on display in our program at Adams State. Denise joined our program right out of high school as a walk-on athlete. She showed some promise and was interested in trying college-level running. In any given year, between 15 and 20 women try out for seven spots to compete at the regional and national meets in November. This means that some really good athletes don't make it.

As the year progressed, so did Denise, and it seemed like she had an outside shot at the seventh and final spot. When the day came to do the final time trail for nationals, Denise was outdistanced by another team member. With her eighth-place finish, she became the alternate for our team. At the national championship, we found ourselves at the top of the pack. Denise was glad to see it, but she wanted to participate. That day she said to me, "That's the last national championship race I plan to watch." The following year, she made the team and placed in the top 25 at the national championships, earning All-American honors and enjoying being on a national championship team as well.

As we headed into the next season, I sat the team leaders down and told them that I had a challenge for them. We had enjoyed tremendous success as a team, but we were lacking in individual champions. I believed that any one of them could win that title and challenged them to train to do it. The next season arrived and it was clear Denise was fit. She had trained hard all summer and made a commitment to do everything right to bring home another team title. She established herself as our team's top runner and was clearly a top runner in the nation at the Division II level. But she had tremendous competition. A school out of Chicago had an older international athlete who came into the national meet undefeated, including racing against some of the top Division I programs.

The night before the Division II meet, the national Athlete of the Year award was given. As the name was called, I could see Denise's disappointment. Her competition had won and she was clearly let down. She approached me and said she was sorry. She had truly wanted that award, not for herself as much as for all the Adams State College women who had deserved it before her. As the tears welled up in her eyes, I looked directly at her and said, "We are not here for the awards they *give* us; we are here for the awards we *earn*. Hold your head up and run that race tomorrow."

As the meet began, I could see Denise's determination. She fought hard and at the 1-mile mark she trailed by about 20 yards. The next phase of the race brought a steep hill; this is where Denise made her move. She caught her competition as they neared the crest of the hill and the rest was history. She poured on the steam and ended up winning the national title with almost a 100-yard lead. As we celebrated at the finish line, we both knew the truth: she had *earned* it.

There are a multitude of great reasons to be motivated to run, and I always go through the benefits and tips that could help my runners stay motivated. Consistency is the key! We all like our routines and feel good when we complete our daily exercise. It's very rewarding to feel that you are improving your health every day.

Other times, running can be somewhat social, and this can be a great impetus to go out for a run. If this is your ticket, then punch it, as your fitness and motivation will both be high. One of the great things about running is you can be one of many or one of a few, or if you prefer a solitary run, that's available as well.

The Human Soul on Fire

Do you lack knowledge or do you lack motivation? As we become smarter about running, health, nutrition, injury prevention, and therapies to recover faster, why do we sometimes not make the right choices? It is important to value what we want, so that the drive "to do" is stronger than the distraction.

I know I sound like a coach, but it is very true. Find what works for you and stick with it. Regardless of whether you just like to look good, or you want to improve your health, or you just love the peace and solitude of a relaxing run, the motivation to stay healthy or come back from injury will be important.

Find your passion; understand the reasons why you are running. Is it because your heart is not as healthy as you want and living a longer life is important? Is it that runner's high and sense of purpose that you have when you finish a run each day? I challenge every runner that I coach to find the reason they do this, and I am challenging you to do the same. When you connect your body, mind, and spirit, then you will know how it feels when the human soul catches fire!

The Least You Need to Know

- Keeping a positive outlook helps you physically.
- If you don't enjoy it, you won't reach goals.
- Motivation is like a vitamin, so take it!
- Running is healthy and relaxing, especially in this era of busy lives.

A

Glossary

ABC drills   These exercises are done to address a different aspect of each running motion, starting with the ankle.

Achilles tendon   This tendon slides through a tube and hooks the two muscles of the calf to the bottom of your heel.

Achilles tendonitis   A classic overuse injury that can also be brought on by adding speed or hill work. *Any* Achilles pain is serious and should be treated as such.

acute injury   The sudden appearance of a new injury, creating pain, which usually means it will take significant time to heal. Never ignore an acute injury.

anemia   When your blood isn't carrying enough oxygen to your muscles, brain, or any part of the rest of your body. Anemia happens most commonly to runners who do not have enough iron in their blood.

antagonistic muscles   Muscles that work in a push-pull action, such as the quadriceps and hamstring in the upper leg, or the triceps and bicep in the upper arm.

athlete's foot   A type of skin disease caused by fungus. If you do get it, most times it appears between your toes first. It commonly attacks your feet because your shoes create the ideal environment (warm and damp) for it to thrive.

biomechanics   The physical properties of proper running.

blisters   Increased stress on the skin as a result of friction or pressure, usually caused by ill-fitting shoes or improper socks.

chafing   What happens when sweating and friction meet. It needs to be addressed immediately, before it leads to wounds and bleeding.

chondromalacia   Also known as "runner's knee," it involves pain under the patella and is often caused by an imbalance of the muscles.

claw toe   Causes toes to stay curled in a "claw" appearance, usually caused by wearing shoes that are too small.

compartment syndrome   A medical condition where increased pressure or swelling in muscle tissues can impair the muscle's ability to do work, including the transportation of blood.

core   Refers to the abs, obliques, and lower back. You need core strength to keep good running form and avoid injuries.

cramps   A sharp, gripping pain in the muscle tissue that can occur because of abnormal fatigue, dehydration, or overheating.

economy of motion   How much force you can use and how to sustain it—finding a balance between the two.

EVA Foam   Ethylene and vinyl acetate (EVA) Foam is widely used in running shoes today to help absorb and lessen the shock of foot strikes while running.

exercise-induced asthma   Symptoms include coughing, wheezing, or chest tightness or chest pain only minutes after you begin running. People with this are very sensitive to temperature and humidity changes.

flexibility   Allows joints to move through a full range of motion.

foot strikes   When the foot hits the ground as you run.

frostbite Can happen to skin and other extremities, particularly those exposed to cold, such as noses, fingers, and so on. Frostbite sneaks up on you—that is, you do not realize it until after it has happened.

hammer toe When a toe folds up permanently at the middle joint.

heat exhaustion A very dangerous condition caused by running in high heat, the body overheating, and improper hydration.

hydration One of the most important aspects of healthy running, it involves drinking enough water and perhaps sports drinks to replace the fluids lost through sweating. Proper hydration is key to avoiding heat-related illnesses.

illiotibial (IT) band A fibrous tissue that runs from the hip over the knee, and attaches just below the knee. It is very susceptible to injury, often from running on the outside of your foot or in shoes that are not a good match for the way you run.

NSAIDs Nonsteroidal anti-inflammatory drugs, such as ibuprofen.

overstriding Taking steps that are too long, which can lead to hamstring and lower leg problems, as well as slower and uneconomical running.

overtorquing This is especially a danger to the hip area, where it causes the upper body to sway back and forth and can lead to tightness in the lower back.

overuse Usually used in the context of "overuse injuries," meaning you have increased your mileage too fast, too soon, or you are training too often, leading to injuries.

periodization Planning your training (running) by dividing your time spent in training into segments with emphasis on developing certain aspects of your running.

plantar fasciitis A severe pain in the fibrous band of tissue that starts at the heel and runs across the bottom of your foot.

polypeptides A chemical released during the hours you are awake, accumulations of which leave you feeling lethargic and unmotivated.

pronation The rolling motion inward of the foot during running.

range of motion   The distances from extension to full contraction. For example, going from an arm bent as much as it can be, to being fully extended.

REM sleep   Rapid eye movement sleep is a period of deep sleep that occurs two to three times each night. REM will usually last 15 minutes every three hours or so of sleep. You can remove polypeptides from your blood during REM sleep.

RICE   Rest, Ice, Compression, and Elevation; this term is used as a prescription for injury treatment and prevention.

sciatica   A horsetail-shaped nerve that comes out of the lower lumbar region, splits at the buttocks area, and continues down both legs, ending at the feet.

shin splints   Pain in the front of the leg, it is often mistaken for bone pain, when in reality shin splints involve irritation of the sheath that surrounds the shin bone.

shuffle   Term used to describe runners who do not have good biomechanics—those who don't lift their heels toward their butt and thus have short, stiff-legged strides without a full range of motion.

side stitch   Pains that are created by the overstretching of ligaments in the abdominal area. The pounding of running while breathing in and out can overstretch these ligaments.

solitude   Something a runner who trains alone can enjoy.

stone bruise   Usually on the bottom of the feet, these contusions are very painful and are often caused by stepping on hard objects.

stress fractures   Not a complete break, but a hairline fracture that takes four to eight weeks to heal, caused usually by chronic trauma and/or poor nutrition. These fractures occur all too often in runners.

sunburn   Caused by overexposure to sun, even in what many would consider only moderate exposure to sunlight; preventable by sunscreen.

supinator   Feet and ankles that roll outward when you run.

supplements   Herbs, vitamins, minerals, and electrolytes that can help aid your body in rest, performance, or recovery.

tight muscles These prevent you from having a full range of motion and can alter your biomechanics, increasing the risk of injury.

trail running Running in the woods, forest, or otherwise off the beaten path, but not necessarily simply a dirt path alongside a concrete or asphalt path. Trails have tree roots, rocks, and other obstacles to be aware of.

trocanteric bursitis A pain between the upper femur and the muscles in that area, caused by the inflammation of bursa sacks in the upper area of the thigh.

vertical oscillation Bouncing up and down as you run. You want to minimize this.

VO2 Max Total amount of oxygen you can take in per minute of exercise divided by your kilograms (2.2 pounds) of bodyweight. This is an important indicator of cardiovascular fitness and performance.

volume In this context, your mileage, or how much you do of something.

windburn This can strip the body's natural oil from the skin, leaving it dried and irritated and giving the skin a "burned" look.

Appendix B

Workouts for Runners at All Levels

Following I have listed a few examples of running programs for the novice runner up to the advanced runner. These programs range from running three to four days a week to running at a more advanced schedule of seven days a week.

Prenovice (Just Getting Started)

Monday: 20 minutes easy running, 5×100-meter strides

Tuesday: OFF

Wednesday: 5 minutes easy warm-up, 15 minutes moderate-to-hard effort, 5 minutes easy cooldown

Thursday: OFF

Friday: 20 minutes easy running, 5×100-meter strides

Saturday: OFF

Sunday: OFF or 25 minutes easy running

Novice (Some Running Experience)

Monday: 25 minutes easy running, 5×100-meter strides

Tuesday: 5 minutes easy warm-up, 20 minutes moderate-to-hard effort, 5 minutes easy cooldown

Wednesday: 30 minutes easy running, 5×100-meter strides

Thursday: OFF

Friday: 25 minutes easy running, 5×100-meter strides

Saturday: OFF

Sunday: 35 minutes easy running

Intermediate

Monday: 35 minutes easy running, 6×100-meter strides

Tuesday: 8 minutes easy warm-up, 25 minutes moderate-to-hard effort, 8 minutes easy cooldown

Wednesday: 40 minutes easy running, 6×100 meter strides

Thursday: OFF

Friday: 10 minutes easy warm-up, dynamic flexibility, 3–4x strides, 3–4x 1,000 meters at 180 bpm heart rate/3–4 minute walk-jog recovery, 10 minutes easy cooldown

Saturday: OFF

Sunday: 60 minutes easy running

Advanced

Monday: 50 minutes easy running, 6×100-meter strides

Tuesday: 10 minute easy warm-up, 25–30 minutes anaerobic threshold run (approximately 170 bpm heart rate), 10 minutes easy cooldown

Wednesday: 55 minutes easy running over hilly terrain

Thursday: 40 minutes easy running, 6×100-meter strides

Friday: 12 minutes easy warm-up, dynamic flexibility, 3–4x strides, 3–4x 1 mile at 180 bpm heart rate/3-minute walk-jog recovery, 12 minutes easy cooldown

Saturday: 40 minutes easy running

Sunday: 70–80 minutes easy running

Appendix C

Resource List

This list includes things I have come across online. These resources should not be substituted for actual medical attention or even self-diagnosis. And although I can't vouch for their accuracy, all in all, what I saw looks pretty good. These websites provide potentially valuable insights.

www.runnersworld.com
A pretty neat and thorough website about running, which includes several dozen sections, many of which deal with running injury-free. This is the website for the hugely popular magazine of the same name.

www.runnersrescue.com
I like this website, because it is dedicated to running injury-free rather than focusing on a time or distance.

www.teamoregon.com/publications/cominjur.html
This web page is unique because it breaks down almost every known running injury, listing probable causes and possible treatments.

www.nismat.org/ptcor/runner
While a lot of websites and periodicals focus on running and even injury-free running, this website gives information primarily on physical therapy as a treatment for runners.

www.injuredrunner.com
Though this website hypes several of its products, it does provide a nice section of terms related to injury-free running.

www.drpribut.com/sports/sportframe.html
This is a blog and website by a podiatrist, covering everything from running in the heat to shoes.

http://orthopedics.about.com/cs/sportsmedicine/a/runninginjury. htm
While many websites focus on specific injuries, this website has information on all kinds of injuries common to runners.

www.podiatrychannel.com/runninginjuries/index.shtml
Again, this website focuses on injury-free running from a podiatry angle, but it also focuses on running injuries and even provides a forum where runners can talk about injuries and see what others have experienced—somewhat akin to what I tried to do in this book with the "In Their Shoes" features.

http://sportsmedicine.about.com/od/runninginjuries/a/ runners_overuse.htm
This is another neat website, because it addresses issues related specifically to overuse, which to me is a constant, even nagging issue for runners seeking to better themselves while avoiding injuries.

http://running.about.com/od/travel/ss/runonvacay.htm
Related to a couple of other websites on this list, this web page actually provides a checklist, as I advised in the book, for runners as to where to run and what to look for when you go on vacation but want to continue running.

www.adams.edu
This is the website for the college at which I teach and coach, Adams State College in Alamosa, Colorado. A pretty cool program and a really great place. Check it out and you'll find my team and me on there somewhere, too!

www.rrca.org
This particular link has great information on clubs, services, coaches, and news related to long-distance running. You will find it valuable if you're looking for support with your own running.

http://runningtimes.com

Running Times magazine provides a great website with training and racing advice, as well as info on shoes and other products. It even has a question-and-answer section where you can ask the experts for advice.

www.usatf.org

This site is run by USA Track and Field, the governing body for long-distance running in America. It has loads of info ranging from rules and anti-doping regulations to current news on American long-distance running.

www.iaaf.org

This site is very similar to the USA Track and Field website, except it is run and maintained by the international governing body. It has loads of info pertaining to rules, regulations, anti-doping, competitions, and so on.

www.runningresearchnews.com

Running Research News produces a monthly newsletter with the latest research about training, nutrition, and sports medicine. This newsletter is very practical and includes articles on how to improve your workouts and prevent injuries.

Index

insoles, 155-156
intake (fluid intake)
  heat-related safety concerns,
    176-177
  supplemental intake, 69-70
  water intake, 68
intensity, training and, 39-41
internal relaxation technique, 134
intrinsic motivation, 245-247
isometrics, strength training programs, 118

J-K-L

jogging strollers, 161-162
journaling, tracking training progress, 35

knees, runner's knee, 213-214

law of reversibility (training), 41-42
law of specificity (training), 42
layering clothing, 156-157
legs
  Front Leg Raise exercise, 121
  injuries and ailments, 214-218
  proper body mechanics, 7
  Side Straight-Leg Raise exercise,
    121
  Straight-Leg Raise exercise,
    121-122
long slow distance training, 53
Lower Back Stretch exercise,
  104-105
lower body
  biomechanics, 6-8
  stretching exercises
    Bent-Leg Hamstring Stretch,
      106
    Foot/Ankle Stretch, 110
    Hamstring/Bench Stretch, 108
    Hamstring Rope/Belt Stretch,
      108
    Hamstring Stretch for the
      Mid-Rear Thigh, 108-109
    Iliotibial Band Stretch, 109

    Lower Calf Stretch, 110
    Lunges, 105-107
    Plantar Fascia Stretch, 111
    Quadriceps Stretch, 109
    Upper Calf Stretch, 110
Lower Calf Stretch exercise, 110
Lunges, 105-107

M

macrocycles, 29
meal-replacement mixes, 69
mechanics
  cooling down, 85
  strength training programs, 118
  stretching, 91-93
medical care options
  active release therapy, 228
  acupuncture, 228
  athletic trainers, 226
  chiropractic care, 227-228
  diet doctors, 226-227
  females, 225
  finding the right provider,
    223-225
  sports psychologist, 227
medicine ball, strength training,
  118-119
mesomorph, 73
microcycles, 29
middle body stretching exercises,
  99-105
  Abdominal Z Stretch, 101
  Back Relaxation—Child Position,
    105
  Cat/Middle Back Stretch, 103
  Glutes Against the Wall, 100-101
  Groin Stretch, 100
  Hip Flexor Stretch, 103-104
  Lower Back Stretch, 104-105
  Reverse Cat/Middle Back
    Stretch, 103
  Waist Stretch, 101-102
motivation issues, 241-247
  finding your passion, 247
  intrinsic versus extrinsic, 245-247

T